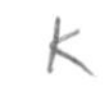

Visions *and* Voices

The Nurse Practitioner Today

Chris Patterson
Editor

To my father,
John Albert Patterson

and

Dr. C. Edward (Ted) Evans
an advocate of NPs who provided countless hours of advice during the development of the NP initiative in Ontario.

First Edition 1997
Second Edition, 1999
ISBN 0-9685510-1-7

1. Nurse Practitioner
2.nursing: Advanced Practice

Published in 1999 by New Grange Press

New Grange Press (Canada), Orkney House, 428 Orkney Road, RR1 Troy, Ontario L0R 2B0, Canada
Telephone: (905) 628-0354, Fax: (905) 628-4901, Internet: idecide@netcom.ca ;
Website: www.netcom.ca/~idecide

New Grange Press (Ireland), The Stables, Woodstown, Waterford, Ireland
Telephone: 353-51-870152, Fax: 353-51-871214

New Grange Press (Australia), Box 7077, Shenton Park, 6008 Western Australia, Australia
Telephone: 61-8-93468107, Fax: 61-8-93468232

New Grange Press (United States),
6600 Harrod's View Circle
Prospect, K.Y. 40059
Telephone: 503 228 2181

Printed in Canada

Acknowledgement

A special thanks to the professional nursing associations across Canada and Dr. Jan Towers, Director of Governmental Affairs, Practice and Research, American Academy of Nurse Practitioners, for their insight into the NP initiative in Canada and the United States. My gratitude to Betty McCarthy, for her secretarial support, Bruno Malibert, for his editorial comments; and to the contributors and other individuals who took time out of their busy schedules to support this project.

Thank you all!

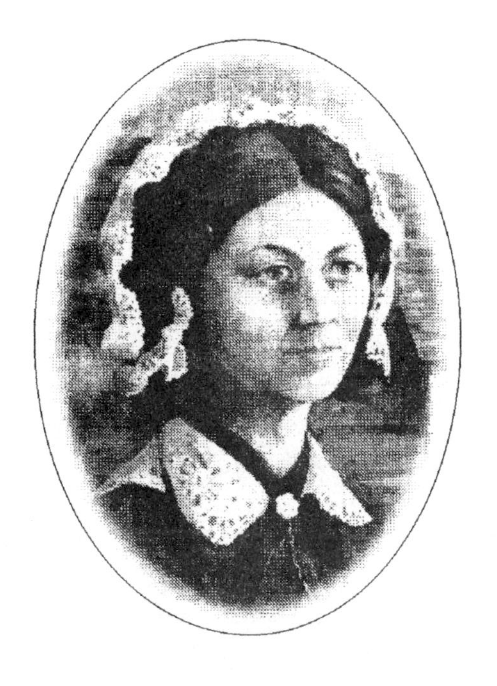

Florence Nightingale
1820-1910
One of the first Advanced Nurse Practitioners

Foreword

Whenever I tell someone that for fifteen years my primary health care provider has been a nurse practitioner, I am usually asked, "What are nurse practitioners and what do they do?" Once that has been explained, the next question is always "Why aren't there more of them?" This book answers both those questions, and makes a valuable contribution to the broader and ongoing debate about the future of Canada's health care system. A debate that is too often focused on how do we pay for health care, rather than on how to get the best value for the money we now spend.

I believe that there is a general consensus that we must change our health care system so that it helps to keep us healthy, as well as treating us when we are ill. There is agreement that this means teaching people to take responsibility for their health, shifting the emphasis from treatment to prevention, and providing a greater range of choices about how we are cared for when we are ill, where we are cared for, and by whom.

There is, however, no consensus about the fundamental issues such changes unleash - issues of money and power, who pays, and how much autonomy do various health professions have. Those are the issues that are central to determining the future of nurse practitioners.

I was very proud as Minister of Health to launch Ontario's nurse practitioner project in February 1994. My objective was to increase the number of nurse practitioners in Ontario, and to establish once and for all their role in the health care system. I have long believed that expanding and clarifying the role of nurse practitioners will be a huge step towards reforming the kind of health care system we have, and making it more cost effective. My experience as Minister only strengthened that conviction.

I am also convinced that dealing with the issues of money and power as they relate to nurse practitioners will set the stage for dealing with those issues in the wider debate about health care. On the other hand, if we cannot agree to expand the role of nurse practitioners, the prospect for real reform of the system is dim.

This book is important to all those interested in the future of health care-providers, payers, and patients. It demonstrates not only the importance of nurse practitioners but contributes to the current debate about fundamental issues of health policy. That is a debate that needs to be joined by all those who believe that Canada's publicly funded and administered health care system must be preserved.

October 3, 1995

Ruth Grier
Ontario Minister of Health
February 1993 - June 1995

Contents

Introduction

A time to reflect...

The nurse practitioner (NP) movement has created a rich history for nursing over the past twenty-five years. In the province of Ontario, this history can be largely attributed to the work of the Nurse Practitioners' Association of Ontario (NPAO), an interest group of the Registered Nurses Association of Ontario (RNAO).

NPAO was founded in 1973 by a group of graduates from the newly established educational programs for nurse practitioners. The purpose of the association was to provide support and networking opportunities for NPs who were returning to a variety of practice settings. These practitioners would begin their new roles in collaborative relationships with physicians. Many would work in primary health care settings, but some would return to secondary and tertiary settings, such as ambulatory care units affiliated with hospitals. The mandate of the NPAO was to develop continuing education programs, and to establish political initiatives to assure the role would continue.

Nurse practitioners reminiscing about these early days of the NPAO called them "heady times." It was not uncommon to have the room filled with high energy during executive meetings. These pioneer practitioners took every opportunity to do television and media interviews to make the role visible. They wrote letters to politicians and nursing leaders to acknowledge the benefits of the NP's role in the health care system. They participated in research studies that were conducted to determine the cost effectiveness, safety, and consumer acceptability for the role.

Nurse practitioners, with advanced knowledge and skills for primary health care, were embarking on a new role in the system. This collaborative role gave nurses the opportunity to make decisions about a client's conditions and recommend therapeutic treatment. It also gave NPs a greater degree of autonomy to use their nursing skills, and participate in health promotion and disease prevention initiatives.

Nurse practitioners were making their mark on the health care system. Even more exciting, NPs were part of the budding health care reform movement that began in the late 1960's and gained momentum during the 1970's and 1980's.

In spite of the findings of studies showing NPs to be cost effective, safe and acceptable to the consumer, the last of the educational programs for nurse practitioners was discontinued in 1983. Politicians had not given the necessary legislative support for expanded role functions. Without legislative support, NPs were unable to order diagnostic tests or prescribe medications for common illnesses. There was no way to reimburse NPs under the fee-for-service system. Lack of appropriate reimbursement mechanisms caused a duplication of service and payment when physicians had to see each patient regardless of the NP's findings. Use of protocols for these activities worked well, but again the approval of physicians was required. The role was becoming more and more unacceptable to physicians. Nursing leaders encouraged that the education for NPs be incorporated into baccalaureate education and withdrew their support from the early educational process. However, nursing leaders continued to support the advanced nursing practice role.

Although the educational programs were discontinued, the NPAO tenaciously continued its efforts to promote the NP's practice and contribution to the health care system. The excitement of the early days was gone, but the vision for NPs working in autonomous primary health care roles persisted. A look at the NPAO's archives revealed continuous efforts to lobby government for the reinstatement of educational programs. It was during these middle years that NPAO recognized the need to strengthen linkages with the RNAO. Brochures were developed, the constitution was revised, and the ongoing dialogue with the Ministry of Health and nursing leaders continued.

By the late 1980's, the health care system was experiencing an economic crisis. Political leaders were now taking the earlier call for health care reform seriously, and with this new orientation to the provision of primary health care, they were reconsidering the role of the nurse practitioner. It was the New Democratic Party (NDP) that announced a plan for the education and employment of nurse practitioners in the 90's.

The Nurse Practitioners' Association of Ontario recognized the need to develop standards of practice. The project began in 1991 and included nurses from numerous sites across the province. The writing of the standards was a dynamic undertaking. The resulting document, Standards of Practice for Nurse Practitioners in Primary Health Care, was published in 1993; it was to become the basis for curriculum development when the new educational programs were reinstated.

With the announced support of the NP's role by the NDP government, the NPAO renewed its lobbying efforts with other nursing organizations. Dorothy Hall was appointed the nursing co-ordinator for the Ministry of Health, Nurse Practitioner Project. She worked tirelessly to bring together nursing leaders from the Registered Nurses Association of Ontario, the College of Nurses of Ontario, the Ontario Nurses Association, and the Nurse Practitioners' Association of Ontario. The result was a strong, united voice from nursing regarding the role. After considerable consultation and negotiation with numerous health care provider groups, nursing groups, and consumer groups, the Ministry of Health announced its plan for the employment and education of NPs.

Since the beginning, there has been a vision for nurse practitioners to work in autonomous roles as full members of an interdisciplinary health care team. The project began with NPs working in primary health care roles, but clearly there is strong evidence that this role is needed and effective in secondary and tertiary settings as well.

The nurse practitioner movement has contributed a richness to nursing history in Canada. The future will see nurses moving into advanced nursing practice roles with opportunities to use their skills and knowledge.

Margaret Snyder, RN, BScN
Past Chairperson,
Nurse Practitioners' Association of Ontario

Contributors

Deb Bisnaire, RN, CNN(C), BNSc, MHSc, Expanded Role Nurse, Division of Neurosurgery, London Health Sciences Centre, University Campus, London, Ontario

Dr. C. Edward Evans, MB, MRSC, FCFP, Family Physician, Family Practice Unit; Professor Department of Family Medicine, McMaster University, Hamilton, Ontario

Anna Giallonardo, RN, MSN, Mental Health Nurse Practitioner, Nurse Educator, Unit One, Queen Street Mental Health Centre, Toronto, Ontario

Shari Glenn, RN, MScN, Nurse Practitioner, North Lanark County Community Health Centre, Lanark, Ontario

Ruth Grier, Ontario Minister of Health, February 1993 - June 1995

Dorothy C. Hall, RN, BSc, MN, LLD, DSc, Past Nursing Coordinator, Ontario Ministry of Health

Bob Harris, RN, MScN, Expanded Role Nurse, Department of Musculoskeletal and Rehabilitation Services, London Health Services Centre, University Campus, London, Ontario

Linda Jones, RN, BScN, Family Nurse Practitioner, South East Ottawa Centre for a Healthy Community, Ottawa, Ontario

Barbara Love, RN, BScN, MHSc, Assistant Professor, School of Nursing, McMaster University; Chairperson of Paediatric Oncology Nursing Program, McMaster University, Hamilton, Ontario

Kathleen MacMillan, RN, BSc, MA (Anthropology) MSc (Nursing), Past President, Registered Nurses Association of Ontario

Barbara Markham, Hons. BSc, MBA, Assistant Coordinator, Centre for Health Economics and Policy Analysis, Department of Clinical Epidemiology and Biostatistics, McMaster University, Hamilton, Ontario

Dorothy-Ann Mills, RN, BN, MHSc, Nurse Practitioner, Family Practice Unit, Chedoke-McMaster Hospitals; Associate Clinical Professor Department of Family Medicine; Associate Member, School of Nursing, McMaster University, Hamilton, Ontario

Johanne Mousseau, RN, BA, MSc, Nurse Practitioner, Assistant Professor, Coordinator of the Northern Clinical Program, McMaster University; Formerly Nursing Consultant for NP Initiative, Ontario Ministry of Health

Dr. Bosco Paes, MD, FRCP (C), FRCP (I), Professor, Department of Paediatrics (Neonatal Division), The Children's Hospital at Chedoke-McMaster Hospitals; Director of Nurseries, St. Joseph's Hospital, Hamilton, Ontario

Leah Parisi, CRNA, BSN, MA, EdD, JD, Professor, School of Nursing, McMaster University, Hamilton, Ontario

Chris Patterson, RN, Hons. BSc (Biology), MScN, Nurse Practitioner, Assistant Professor, School of Nursing, McMaster University, Hamilton, Ontario

Janet Pinelli, RNC, MScN, DNS, Associate Professor, School of Nursing, McMaster University; Clinical Nurse Specialist/Neonatal Practitioner, Chedoke-McMaster Hospitals, Hamilton, Ontario

Rita Schreiber, RN, DNS, Assistant Professor, School of Nursing, University of Victoria, Victoria, BC

Margaret Snyder, RN, BScN, Nurse Practitioner, Past Chairperson, Nurse Practitioners' Association of Ontario, 1994-96

Karen Titanich, RN, MScN, MPH, Principal, Vital Connections™ , Edmonton, Alberta; Formerly Project Manager Workforce Planning Branch, Alberta Health, Edmonton, Alberta

Dr. Daniel Way, MD, CCFP, Family Physician, South East Ottawa Centre for a Healthy Community; Assistant Professor, Department of Family Medicine, University of Ottawa, Ottawa, Ontario

Susanne Williams, RN, BNSc, MEd, Professor and Director, School of Nursing, Ryerson Polytechnic University, Toronto, Ontario

Chapter One

Nurse Practitioners in Canadian Health Care
We're Not Out of the Woods Yet!

Chris Patterson,
Janet Pinelli,
Barbara Markham

The nurse practitioner's (NP) role has been the topic of academic, professional, and political discussions for some time in both Canada and the United States. In contrast to their American colleagues, the progress of the NP in Canada has not been as successful. In fact, the history of the NP movement in Canada can be compared more to a phenomenon waiting to be rediscovered than a progressive integration of the role into the health care system. For Ontario and Alberta NPs, the role has been revived, historically marking this as a period of intense activity, a milestone in the evolution of the role.

Canadian NPs: Lost in the Woods or Slow to Find the Way?

The nurse practitioner movement in both Canada and the United States began in the mid-1960s. In 1965, the first NP program was established in the U.S. with the goal of expanding the role of the nurse for the delivery of health care to well children and their families.[1,2] It was not until 1967 that the first educational program for NPs in Canada was started at Dalhousie University, in Nova Scotia. Eventually, several programs in Canada were established to educate nurses to work in northern communities, but these programs were stopped in 1983 because of a perceived oversupply of physicians, reimbursement issues, lack of legislation and lack of public awareness of the role.[3]

The aborted efforts for establishing NPs in Canada has resulted in a sharp decline in the number and level of educational programs for NPs in Canada in contrast with those of the United States. In the U.S., there are currently 190 institutions with master's level NP programs, with 97 more institutions planning to initiate graduate and post-master's certificate programs.[4] In 1992, more than 80% of programs preparing NPs were at the graduate level, with only women's health care having any significant number of non-master's programs.[5] Currently, there are very few certificate programs, with the majority still in women's health.[A] Thus, in addition to the large number of educational programs available to educate NPs, the greatest percentage of U.S. federally funded programs today are at a master's level.[6] In fact, non-federally funded educational programs are also tending towards master's preparation for NPs.[B] By comparison, there are few programs in Canada that are specifically designed to prepare NPs. As of September 1995, Ontario was the only province to offer a provincial educational program to educate NPs at a baccalaureate level for primary health care.[C] In 1997, Athabasca University offered an advanced graduate diploma in community nursing practice, which prepares graduates for expanded nursing roles. In Quebec, the University of Sherbrooke offers a graduate diploma program in nursing sciences which prepares advanced practice nurses; a master's program encompassing the present diploma program is being developed. Educational preparation for acute care NPs is limited to three programs offered at McMaster University, the University of Toronto, and the University of Alberta.[D] . As well, there are a few programs in Canada educating nurses for expanded roles. These programs are situated in universities and colleges in Nova Scotia, Ontario, and Saskatchewan.[7] In the Northwest Territories, the Department of Health and Social Services offers an advanced nursing skills in-service program to prepare nurses practising in the community. In addition to formal training programs, there are ad hoc attempts by administrators to train nurses for expanded roles in hospital settings.

NPs in the U.S. have made important inroads. Development of reimbursement mechanisms, recognition by professional colleagues, establishment of national certifying bodies and regulation of practice by state boards of nursing, development of professional organizations and obtainment of prescriptive authority are but a few of the gains made by NPs in the United States over the last several years. In the U.S., nurse practitioners, clinical nurse specialists, nurse midwives, and nurse anaesthetists are recognized as advanced practice nurses (APNs). In a state by state review of the legislative, legal, prescriptive authority, and reimbursement status for APNs (which included NPs), Pearson (1995) noted:

> In several states APNs do not yet have full state legislative authority to diagnose and treat; yet even within the most restrictive of these states, the barriers are beginning to break down. In virtually no state are the legislative practice restrictions making a trend toward becoming more restrictive.[8]

As of April 1997, Canadian NPs have not been successful in obtaining legislation to support expanded role activities - except for Alberta-despite the fact that the NP movement in both countries began at approximately the same time. In 1996, registered nurses' associations in Canada were contacted by one of the authors (Chris Patterson) to determine the current location of NPs and the perceived future of the NP role. Since there has been no formal mechanism in place for registration or certification of NPs as in the U.S., the number of NPs employed in Canada could not be obtained. However, in 1994, the best estimate was that approximately 250 nurses in Ontario are practising as NPs.[9] In provinces where nurses work in expanded roles, they are situated mostly in outpost stations, isolated areas or clinics. For example, in Newfoundland, regional nurses work in areas of northern Newfoundland and Labrador where individuals have limited access to medical service. These nurses perform many of the expanded role functions traditionally associated with the NP model in Ontario, such as diagnosing, prescribing, and treating. A similar situation exists in Saskatchewan, the Northwest Territories, Yukon, Manitoba, New Brunswick, and British Columbia. In some provinces, expanded role nurses may use the title NP; however, diversity among their educational preparations exists. Presently, there is no legislation to support the current expanded practice of these nurses. These responsibilities remain under the delegation of physicians; and, nurses may practise under physician-approved protocols.

How the roles of the NP and the registered nurse (RN) will develop in the future are being discussed in Canada within a climate of change, created by health care reform and shrinking health care dollars. Much of the political activity about the role of the NP in the Canadian health care system has been located in Ontario and Alberta. Both the Ontario Ministry of Health and Alberta Health began a systematic process to investigate mechanisms for more effective use of NPs. Although it is difficult at this time to predict the degree to which the NP will be established in Canada, it appears that the potential remains for a more expanded role for nurses.

We began this chapter by comparing the current status of NPs in the U.S. and Canada, and the differences between the two countries in securing support for expanded role activities. Adjusting for population, Canada has approximately 7.5% the number of NPs compared to the U.S.[E] Why has the NP movement in the United States been more successful than in Canada? We believe that there are at least three important reasons:

1. differences between countries in terms of health care funding sources;
2. the organization of NPs; and
3. a certain level of political will within governments to allow NPs to make inroads into the legislative process.

Funding Source and Delivery Differences Between Canada and the US: Divergent Paths

The growth of health care industry expenditures in the U.S. has significantly outpaced the growth of expenditures in Canada when measured against Gross Domestic Product.[11] (Graph #1)

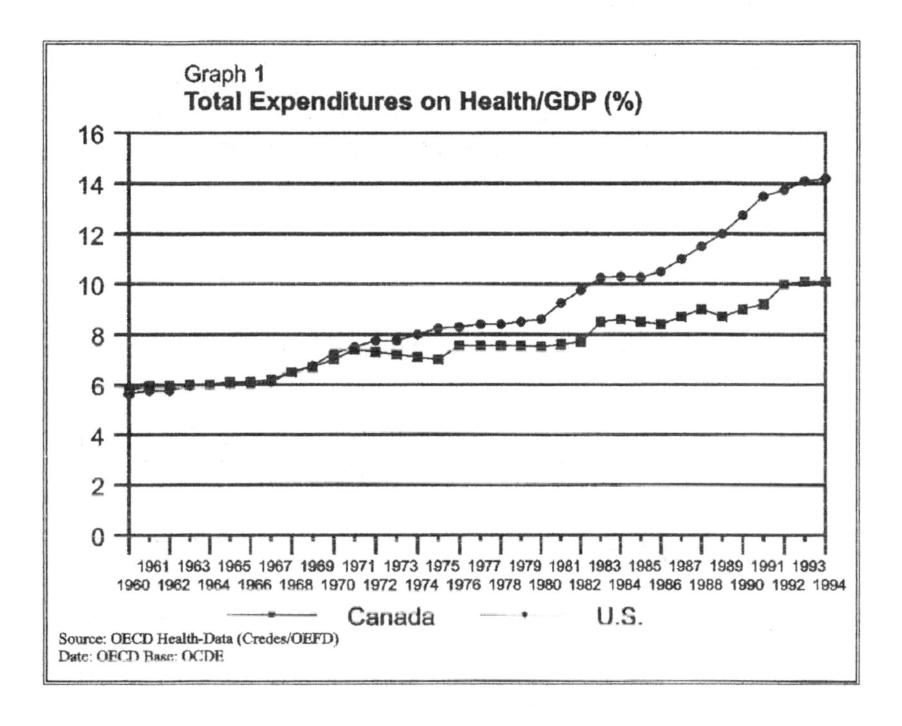

This has led some analysts to conclude that cost containment efforts in the U.S. have failed relative to efforts in Canada and other countries.[12,13] With the demise of the recent Clinton health reform initiatives, we can predict that the U.S. and Canada will continue on their divergent expenditure paths for the foreseeable future.

One suggested reason for higher health care expenditures in the U.S. compared to Canada is the difference in funding arrangements. The fragmentation of funding sources in the largely private and competitive U.S. health care market is thought to have fostered the relatively large expansion in health expenditures.[13] In contrast, Canada raises revenue for health expenditures primarily through the public sector. This sole source funding appears to be a critical success factor for cost control.[12] For example, we note from Graph #1 the divergence in expenditures between the U.S. and Canada in the early 1970s, only three years after the introduction of Medicare in Canada.

The pattern for overall health expenditures is also reflected in physician service expenditures. Increasing physician expenditures are due to increasing physician numbers per capita population (Graph #2) and increasing average physician incomes.[11] (Graph #3)

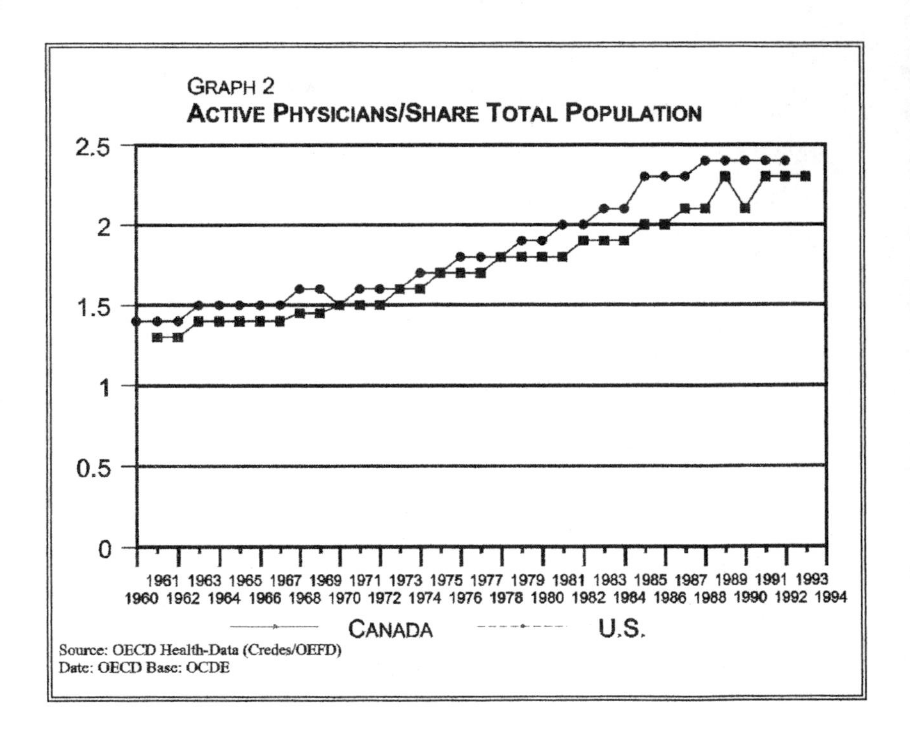

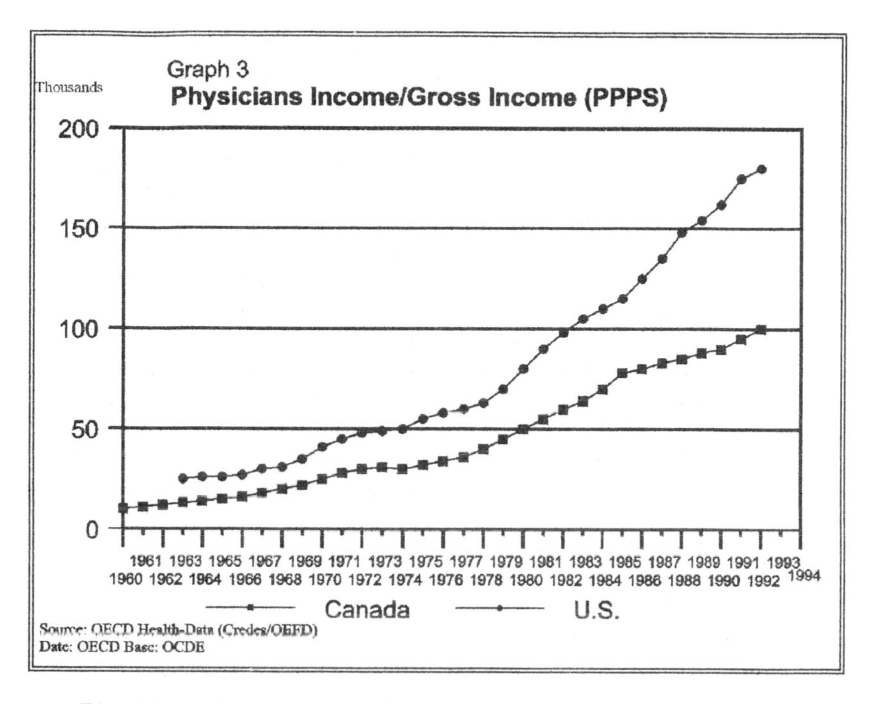

Physician expenditures in Canada have been constrained, in part, by government-controlled increases to provincial physician fee schedules (control of price). The quantity of physician services is constrained to some extent through global budget funding of hospitals.[F] However, these price and quantity control measures are limited since the vast majority of Canadian physicians are paid on a fee-for-service basis. Such a system is open-ended in that physicians are free to increase services to keep pace with their income expectations. Additionally, since new physicians are free to set up practice in their chosen location and bill their respective provincial health care system, Canadian governments have no effective policy levers to ensure an equitable geographical distribution of physician resources.[G] In Canada, as in the U.S., the supply of new physicians has continued to outpace population growth, causing unrelenting upward pressure on expenditures. The ability of Canadian governments to cope with increased health care expenditures, however, has been weakened by two deep and protracted recessions in the last decade. Thus, it has been increasingly viewed by policymakers that we are spending too much on health care, and that this is caused in large part by an oversupply of physicians.[14] Health human resource substitution is much less likely to occur in times and areas of perceived physician surplus. [15]

As long as physicians in Canada are paid fee-for-service, the introduction of NPs will be viewed as an "add-on" in terms of cost to the system,[16] even though evidence has shown that the introduction of NPs has the potential to reduce system expenditures. The NP can perform many of the services of a physician (estimates range between 40 to 90%), at the same or higher quality and patient acceptance, and for a reduced cost. They also tend to be less intensive users of system resources.[17,18] However, under the present fee-for-service system, physician services displaced by the NP can reappear as increased services in other areas as physicians seek to replace lost income. Without additional controls on physician expenditures, overall system expenditures would likely increase with the addition of more NPs. Thus, under the current organizational and funding arrangements in Canada, there is unlikely to be an overall system expenditure saving with the introduction of NPs, and as Spitzer has noted, this has led to the slow death of a good idea.[16,19,20]

Although large changes in the accepted role of the NP in Canada must await physician payment reform, smaller inroads continue to be made in underserviced regions such as rural areas, the North and inner-city slums, in specialties like obstetrics and gynaecology and neonatal care,[10] and in the care of homeless populations. It has been noted that the NP role originated, in part, in response to the need for basic medical services in inner-city and rural areas which were underserved by physicians.[21]

It is sometimes argued that increasing physician specialization has led to increased utilization of NPs, and there is some evidence for this when comparing Canada and the U.S. It is difficult to compare countries because of differences in classification;[H] however, it is generally accepted that there are proportionally more specialist physicians in the U.S. compared to Canada. In addition, access to specialists in Canada is more difficult as it requires a referral.

One aspect of the U.S. health care system which has supported the introduction of large numbers of NPs has been the introduction of managed care organizations such as Health Maintenance Organizations (HMOs). An increasing proportion of the U.S. population belongs to managed care settings.

These organizations are unique in that physician staff are paid by salary. NPs hired into such an environment have the potential to replace physician services and reduce costs overall. The Canadian equivalent, such as Community Health Centres (CHCs), covers a much smaller percentage of the population. Increased pressures from large businesses and insurers to reduce health care costs provide conditions for the growth of HMOs and for alternative funding of lower-cost substitute personnel such as NPs.[23] In fact, it is predicted that an increasing number of NPs will be employed in managed care settings in the U.S. in the future.[i]

Physician opposition can be a barrier to the entry of the NP. While physician groups in both countries have always opposed the introduction of NPs, this opposition is becoming louder from physicians in U.S. HMOs[j] and from physicians in Canada, especially in Ontario, where there have been recent moves to reintroduce NPs. More organized physician opposition may be due in part to the recent introduction of cost-containment policies in Ontario (i.e., physician expenditure caps), which place physicians in more direct competition with NP services for scarce health care dollars. We would predict opposition to NPs would be greater in Canada compared to the U.S. because physician interests are more concentrated in Canada and may be in a better position than their U.S. counterparts to prevent or inhibit the introduction of the NP. It is also the case that average physician incomes in the U.S. are high relative to other countries and growing. Without significant expenditure controls, it may be that many perceive there are enough health care dollars to support both physicians and alternative health personnel. Indeed, there are fewer nurses per capita than in Canada, and it may even be viewed that there is a nursing shortage, further supporting expenditures on NPs.[23] As long as NPs do not compete directly with physicians (e.g., they continue to enter practice primarily in areas that are being abandoned by physicians), they will not be perceived as a threat by the vast majority of U.S. physicians.

It has been argued that differences in the funding and organization of health systems in the U.S. and Canada are rooted in deep political, philosophical, and cultural differences.[13] Some of these differences may help to explain the relative success of U.S. NPs compared to Canadian NPs in getting supporting legislation for expanded roles in diagnosing and prescribing. It may be that, in the U.S., free markets in health care services are more likely to support the introduction of health personnel substitutes through the necessary legislative changes. Many U.S. states have undertaken the changes necessary to allow NPs to legally substitute for certain physician-regulated services. In Canada, there has been no province that has supported the legislative changes to legalize NP substitution, except for Alberta. However, on April 30, 1997, the first reading of the *Expanded Nursing Services for Patients Act* which amends the *Nursing Act* and other related acts that allow primary health care NPs to communicate a diagnosis, prescribe and administer certain treatments and medications, and order certain ultrasounds, x-rays and lab tests, was announced by the Honourable Jim Wilson, Ontario Minister of Health. The Act is expected to be proclaimed in the fall of 1997.

In this section, we have argued that differences in funding and health care delivery models have provided more opportunities for NPs to break health care industry barriers in the U.S. compared to Canada. This is in spite of similar concerns about physician surpluses among policymakers. U.S. legislative structures, which reflect a value for private competition in health care, have also provided the necessary legislation to support NPs as legal substitutes who provide some physician services.

In the next section, we look at the organization of nurses as a contributing factor to differences between countries.

Organization of Nurses and Political Will to Make Changes

In the early 1970s, in the U.S., there was a need for expanded nursing roles and a recognition that most state nursing acts restricted nurses from assuming these new roles.[24] Idaho became the first state to take the step-although under careful scrutiny of the Board of Medicine and Idaho State Board of Nursing-towards recognizing statutorily that diagnosis and treatment are within the scope of practice of advanced nurse practitioners or specialty nurses.[24] Although almost all states have legally acknowledged to some degree the expanded role of NPs,[24,8] national legislation to support all advanced practice roles, including the role of the NP, failed with Clinton's health care reform plan.[8] Regardless of the restrictions that still exist in state and national statutes, there has been a certain amount of political will in the United States to allow NPs to achieve a considerable level of success in chipping away at practice barriers. As we have already seen, except for recent initiatives in Ontario and Alberta, there has been little political action taken by provincial governments in Canada to legally support expanded roles to any degree, regardless of the perceived need to reform primary health care and control health care costs.

Another factor influencing the legislative progress of NPs in the two countries has been the critical mass of NPs. A certain critical mass is required to maintain momentum in the political process. Although there are concerns about divisiveness among the many alliances and coalitions fragmenting advanced practice nurses' power,[8] there is organization at the national and state level, as well as a large number of 'grass root' NPs, to lobby for change.

A different situation exists in Canada. Although the Nurse Practitioners' Association of Ontario has promoted and lobbied for NPs, there is no national group to co-ordinate efforts and organize NPs in Canada. Lack of protection of the title has allowed nurses to use the term 'NP' freely, creating more confusion within the ranks. In addition, the nursing profession is still deliberating as to the nature of advanced practice and the 'medical overtones' of the NP model. Compared to the U.S., the NP movement in Canada is still fragmented and has yet to begin to form the necessary structure for developing a power base.

The Re-emergence of the NP Model in Ontario and Alberta: A Clearing in the Woods

At certain periods in time, political and economic forces can combine in such a way as to create opportunities for growth in a profession. An analysis of these forces within a particular environmental context can provide us with insights into how professional roles are shaped. To better understand the renewed interest in the role, a summary of the complex interplay of political and economic pressures that have simultaneously encouraged and constrained the demand for this role is provided.

In 1994, Ruth Grier, the Minister of Health in Ontario, announced a plan for the ongoing education and employment of NPs as equal partners in multidisciplinary health care teams and also as independent practitioners. It was seen at this time that the priority placement of NPs would be in primary health care settings, leaving the potential role of NPs in secondary and tertiary care placements a consideration for future discussions.

Initially, the plan was to exempt nurse practitioners from the prohibition on performing specific controlled acts with the intent of possibly opening the *Nursing Act* at the earliest opportunity to formalize the expansion of nursing practice.[25] Amendment to the *Nursing Act* would consolidate the advanced clinical activities into a newly defined scope of practice for NPs. The Health Professions Regulatory Advisory Council (HPRAC) did not recommend exemption as the most appropriate route on the existing evidence, and requested further information before a decision would be made. It was not until 1996, that HPRAC finally made recommendations to the Minister of Health supporting the expanded role of NPs.[26]

Currently, even though the decision has been made in Ontario to consider only generalists in primary health care, there is considerable interest for extending this to specialist NPs in secondary and tertiary care settings. As well, one may make the argument for the need for NPs whose practice is defined by an age group or a focus in a particular area in primary health care (e.g. gerontology). Presently, there is no commonly accepted definition within the nursing profession for specialist NPs. If the title of NP is protected in the future, recognition of specialist NPs should be considered since they also perform the additional controlled acts under delegation.

In May 1995, after consultation with stakeholders, amendments to the *Alberta Public Health Act* were completed to enable nurses to provide extended health services. Under this Act, nurses are able to diagnose and treat common illnesses of adults and children, refer clients, and provide emergency services. Regional health authorities in Alberta will be able to determine the use of registered nurses who provide extended services, subject to regulations.[K]

These nurses are referred to as 'registered nurses providing extended services' rather than 'nurse practitioners.' The term nurse practitioner is most often associated with physician substitution, whereas registered nurses in Alberta provide nursing services and extended services within the context of nursing. The Alberta Association of Registered Nurses (AARN) is presently examining how registered nurses who provide extended services will be regulated.[K]

The AARN believes that the provision of extended health services must not be confused with advanced nursing practice or an expanded role for registered nurses. Advanced nursing practice is seen as practice where nursing services are offered beyond the basic level as a consequence of the nurse's additional experience, education, and skills.[27] Advanced nursing practice could include, for example, initiating a health promotion counselling program for homeless families, participating on a multidisciplinary committee to develop a national strategy to reduce the incidence of family violence, or coordinating the nursing care for multisystem failure trauma patients. Advanced nursing practice implies that the services provided are within the scope of nursing practice as defined by the Nursing Practice Standards[28] and are performed at the expert level. Registered nurses providing extended health services may or may not be practising at an advanced nursing level.[L]

Nurses providing extended health services will require at a minimum three to five years of experience as a registered nurse, a baccalaureate degree in nursing and completion of an approved program that prepares them to provide extended health care services. Collaboration with other health professionals, especially physicians and pharmacists, and participation as a member of an interdisciplinary team are essential components in the practice of nurses providing these services.[M]

Changing Frameworks and Priorities: NPs in the Context of Health Care Reform

Prior to the 1970s, it appeared to be implicitly accepted that the best way to improve the health of a population was to enhance the availability and sophistication of diagnostic technology and curative medical treatments. In both Canada and the U.S., there has been a rapid expansion in numbers of physicians, hospital beds, pharmaceutical, and new diagnostic and therapeutic technologies. Until recently in some countries, the thrust for increased curative health care has consumed an ever-increasing proportion of national resources. Yet despite this massive build-up of curative medical technologies, human and capital resources, we have not seen commensurate improvements in the general health of society.[29] The medical model cannot be the only model of service delivery.

Since at least the early 1970s, and with support from the influential Lalonde Report,[30] there has been increasing recognition and acceptance by the public and policymakers that societal health and well-being may be more dramatically influenced by determinants of health outside of the curative care industry.[29] Evidence continues to build that employment, socioeconomic status, lifestyles, and safe and supportive environments are more important factors influencing health than simply curative care. This changed and broadened conceptualization of the determinants of health has, in part, resulted in recent policy attempts to shift some health care resources from curative to health promotion efforts.

The term 'health promotion' had been around for some time before it gained more formal recognition with health promotion initiatives of the federal government such as the Lalonde Report, Achieving Health for All: A Framework for Health Promotion and the Ottawa Chapter for Health Promotion.[31] As one may have expected, there has not been a nationally accepted consensus as to the best approach to health promotion.[32] Whether or not the movement of health promotion has reached its full potential, there has been a gradual shift in thinking towards a more expanded concept of health and wellness care, both nationally and internationally.

Why has this movement toward a more expanded concept of health been so important to nursing? It is because the professional orientation of nursing revolves around concepts of individual, family or community, health and the environment. These concepts drive not only the philosophical beliefs of the profession but educational curricula and the diverse practices of nurses, making their expertise potentially valuable to health promotion efforts. Mitchell, Pinelli, Patterson and Southwell (1993) note:

> To optimize the expertise of the nurse, the setting should provide services beyond the traditional medical model to include management of non-medical influences on health, a holistic approach to illness and its impact on quality of life issues, commitment to health promotion and maintenance, and a continued interest in planning care on the needs of the community.[3]

Historically, nursing has been committed to promoting health from a clinical perspective and advocating for health promotion at a political level. Nurses' holistic approach to health and illness makes it easy for them to accept and support health promotion initiatives and to take an active leadership role in the health promotion movement within Canada.

Employers (or at least those involved in primary care) and planning bodies also seem to recognize and accept a health promotion role for nurses. The findings of a needs assessment completed by McMaster University, in collaboration with the Health Human Resources Branch in Ontario, suggested that, among the participating agencies, NPs were cited as potential providers in unmet health promotion and illness-related issues in the community.[33] Study respondents from primary care agencies and planning bodies in the province were asked to identify unmet services in the community and the need for NP services among individuals and families with limited access to health care in Ontario. Of the top 20 unmet needs identified by primary care agencies and planning bodies, 13 are common to both: health promotion/disease prevention services, well baby care, psychiatric services, well women care, reproductive health care, health services for specific illnesses, health education for aggressive behaviour and cognitive impairment, access to medical facilities and clinics, drug and alcohol abuse rehabilitation and detoxification centres, counselling and crisis management for all age groups, adolescent health care, primary health care and social services.[33]

A Growing Awareness of the Use of Non-Physician Substitutes

NPs have been quick to point out that their education and placement makes them well-suited for an expanded role in Canada's changing health system. Numerous studies have found that NPs not only provide quality, cost-effective service but also found consumers to be satisfied with the care they received.[3] Despite the evidence to support the NP's role, NPs remain underutilized.

Underutilization of NPs is recognized by non-nurses as well. In 1991, Barer and Stoddart were commissioned by the Federal/Provincial/Territorial Conference of Deputy Ministers of Health to prepare a discussion paper on physicians' resource management problems. The objectives of this comprehensive report were to determine the perception and extent of agreement on the main problems and issues across Canada about physician resources, and to develop solutions and policy avenues.[14] Although many issues and priority problems were identified that related to medical resource policies, there were a number of recommendations throughout the document related to the use of non-physician personnel. These recommendations had particular importance not only for nurse practitioners but health care providers in general in which there has been evidence to suggest their competence in the delivery of services.

Considerations in Role Development: Seeing the Forest or Simply the Trees

Future challenges remain for nursing educators, professional nursing organizations, and nurses in Canada. Many of these challenges are derived from the continued development of the NP in the U.S. To stimulate thought on issues of advanced practice nursing, we have capitalized on the American experience in order to draw conclusions as to future considerations for developing the role of the Canadian NP. The variability of educational programs and level of preparation, portability of practice, scope of practice issues, NP integration into the health care system, consumer awareness and acceptance of the role, and professional advocacy and lobbying are discussed below.

The Potential Threat of Variability within Educational Programs

The variability within educational programs in the U.S. has raised questions regarding the continued quality of NP preparation and the ability to maintain standards for credentialing of NPs.[34] The strength of the educational initiative within Ontario is the development of a provincial standardized curriculum to prepare NPs and the evaluation of the effectiveness of the program. If educational institutions in other provinces develop programs for NPs, nursing leaders should consider establishing national standards for curriculum development to avoid the inconsistencies found in the U.S. Currently, in the U.S., the major NP organizations are working with NP faculties to establish curriculum standards and a national system of accreditation for NP educational programs.[34]

Master's Preparation for Entry into Advanced Practice

In the U.S., the movement toward master's preparation was influenced by the acceptance of the role by university faculties, increases in federal funding for education, and an expressed need for more advanced educational preparation by NPs.[5] It is likely that a similar movement toward master's education will eventually occur in Canada. The complexities of health care, the movement toward community-based services, the autonomous nature of the NP's decision-making, the demands of technology, and the need for evidence-based practice will create the push toward a higher level of preparation. Educators and practitioners should be involved in ongoing evaluation of educational programs, identification of the appropriate level of education to fulfil expected role responsibilities, and discussion with the government on scope of practice and funding.

A Mechanism for Credentialing to Allow Freedom of Movement within Canada and to Ensure Competencies of NPs

In the U.S., the definition of NP arose from state laws which regulated practice. The first state, Idaho, determined that NP practice should be regulated by policies and procedures (protocols) written at the local level.[5] Other approaches that supported NP practice included the broadening of the definition of registered nurses and the movement by some states to give physicians more delegative powers. The final approach used in the U.S. to accommodate expanded nursing functions was to use the regulatory power of the state to separately certify or license advanced practice nurses. This approach provides for a separate title for advanced practitioners and a defined scope of function for their actions. Currently, the vast majority of states in the U.S. have defined and authorized the role of the NP through such practice acts. In the remaining states, NPs are authorized by an expanded registered nurse statute, by permitting protocols or by allowing physicians more delegating authority.[5]

In the U.S., the definition of a NP from a legal perspective, therefore, depends upon the state in which the NP practises. This definition includes eligibility requirements, as well as delineation of role implementation. It includes a range of advanced practice nurses, as well as practice settings. Requirements for licensure include graduation from a recognized educational program and credentialing from a professional organization. Restricted movement from state to state among NPs is due to the lack of standardization among regulatory boards.

In order to avoid the regulatory problems which have occurred in the U.S., Canadian nursing professional and regulatory bodies need to address the following issues:

1. the value of standardizing educational programs and offering national certification which would be accepted by all provincial regulatory bodies;
2. unrestricted movement of NPs across provinces by the recognition of common certification with a universal title; and
3. the establishment of clinical specialty certification in advanced nursing practice versus role certification as a NP or CNS.

The Importance for Legal Recognition of Expanded Role Activities

Without legal recognition to perform activities currently legislated to medicine, NPs' practice will be restricted. Leaders of the NP movement must continue, therefore, to address the issues of prescriptive authority and diagnosing. The decision remains as to whether to continue to fight for unlimited diagnosing and prescriptive authority or to compromise, which would delineate a more limited scope of practice. However, unlimited diagnosing and prescriptive authority would allow the flexibility for NPs working in primary, secondary or tertiary care settings to function within their different practices without making legislative changes for each type of NP. By restricting prescribing and diagnosing, certain NPs would be excluded until the necessary legislation is passed; furthermore, NPs would be restricted to performing only what the legislation describes even if out of date.

Integration of the Role into the Health Care System

From our perspective, the meaning of independence is more than establishing one's own practice within a community or institution. It is the ability to make independent decisions and to act on behalf of the patient, to provide safe and expedient care within an accepted scope of practice. However, independence in NP practice has been perceived as encroaching on other professionals' territories without adequate knowledge and skills when it is really related to power and economics. If we are to witness enhanced integration of the NP role, nursing organizations must lobby for appropriate human resource management which allows for services to be given by the most appropriate and cost-effective provider. These strategies include financial incentives and disincentives, physician payment reform, and other health care delivery reform initiatives.

Educating the Consumer to the Role and Use of Different Providers

Generally , the NP movement has never had significant consumer support. Because of the small number of NPs in Canada, the public exposure to the care NPs provide has been limited. As well, the Canadian public has been socialized into a medical model of care, thereby reducing their awareness of alternative models. The contributions of medicine to the health care system cannot be minimized; however, the value of other providers and different ways of healing must be publicized and fully realized. It is an essential and immediate task for all NPs and professional nursing organizations to mount public education campaigns demonstrating the ability of nurses and NPs to improve patient health and well-being.[3] We have learned from our American colleagues that consumer support is a powerful ally against medical domination in the health care system.

Political Involvement of Professional Organizations and Practitioners

Another factor for successful implementation of the role in the U.S. has been the ability of NPs to organize politically and continually monitor and react to legislative barriers to NPs' practice. In order to be credible, NPs must be able to clearly articulate who they are and what difference they make to the health care system as nurses and not simply physician/resident replacements. The changes that have occurred through the efforts of 'grass root' NPs and professional American nursing organizations have provided an excellent example of the importance for all NPs to be involved in the legislative process.[35] It will only be through the commitment of NPs and nursing bodies in Canada that the necessary changes will occur.

Multiple Titles for Advanced Nurse Practitioners

Multiple titles for advanced practice nurses at the state level create confusion within the profession, government and other payers, among the public, and other professionals. There exists in the U.S. multiple levels of specialty credentialing and role delineation. For example, a RN with the required number of practice hours in a specialty can apply for specialty certification. This certification is different from a graduate of an NP program seeking certification as a specialist NP. The latter involves an advanced practice component.

Several provincial/territorial nursing associations in Canada have expressed concerns regarding the many different titles given to nurses performing functions within the scope of practice of the NP. Different titles for nurses practising in the expanded role have caused consumer confusion[36] and have created subpopulations of clinicians, making regulation difficult.[5] In 1995, the Nurse Practitioners' Association of Ontario released a position statement regarding title protection. They endorsed "the position that the title of Nurse Practitioner (NP) be a protected title and registered with the College of Nurses under the Extended Class..."[37]

The differences and similarities between clinical nurse specialists and nurse practitioners have received a considerable amount of attention. Within the literature, authors have addressed the similarities and uniqueness of the two roles. Hanson (1990) reported that the differences between the two roles have blurred as NPs and CNSs have crossed into different settings. However, Martin (1990) stated that differences in their functions exist regardless of the setting, with CNSs focusing on acute illness and NPs on health promotion, illness prevention, and management of chronic stable conditions.[38] Elder and Bullough (1990) stated that "...although there are some different tasks carried out by members of the two groups and although they tend to use different terms to describe their diagnostic practices, the large area of overlapping functions and opinions on professional issues is the most impressive finding of the study."[39] Fenton and Brykczynki (1993) reported that "... there is evidence that there is an advanced practice role for both the CNS and the NP and that much of the knowledge, skills and competencies are shared depending on the setting and the clinical situation. There is also evidence that there are distinct differences and emphases for both roles."[40]

Although it is not the intention to settle this debate, it is important to highlight that different titling of advanced practice nurses is an important professional issue, as well as how we regulate different levels of nursing practice. It is essential that nurses define advanced nursing practice so that future research on expanded roles can be guided by an advanced nursing practice model. This will allow insight into not only nurses' abilities to perform certain services traditionally performed by medicine but also their contribution as advanced nurse practitioners to the health care system.

Conclusion

The nature of the Canadian health care system, lack of legislation for all expanded roles, and lack of organization of NPs are major factors slowing the implementation of the role. Despite the restrictions, NPs continue to practice in a legal grey zone. The message is clear, at least to us. The debate is not whether NPs are capable practitioners as demonstrated through a multitude of research studies, but whether the government and public have the will to support the use of other health providers in health care reform. Appropriate educational programs and employment opportunities, professional standards, reimbursement mechanisms, and legislation are all necessary preconditions for establishing an effective NP role. Without these supports, NPs will never find their way toward acceptance and integration in the Canadian health care system.

Chapter 2

Are Nurse Practitioners Contributing to the Growth of the Nursing Profession?

Chris Patterson

In the U.S., nurse practitioners are under the umbrella of advanced nursing practice. The influence from our American colleagues would make it easy for nurses in Canada to equate a NP's role with 'advanced nursing practice.' However, no consensus among nursing leaders has been reached, to date, in most provinces or nationally as to whether this role is advanced nursing practice. Part of the professional hesitation can be related to the lack of clarity as to what constitutes advanced practice[1] and uncertainty about the direction that role expansion in nursing should take in Canada. For these reasons, important political and professional issues for the next decade will be to determine an accepted definition of advanced nursing practice, professional standards, educational requirements and legislation to support the role, as well as its interface with the rest of nursing.

Since the professional definition of advanced nursing practice remains vague in Canada, NPs are generally referred to as having an expanded practice. Mass (1995) noted that "Expanded practice means that, in addition to providing nursing care, nurses perform functions that are within the legislated, or conventionally accepted, scope of practice of another profession."[2] Because NPs perform expanded role functions legislated to medicine, there may be a tendency to conceptualize the role into nursing and medical components. However, in reality, the expanded role functions and the knowledge to competently perform them are blended into nursing practice. NPs not only assess health and illness issues but determine their impact on the spiritual, psychosocial, and functional aspects of the individual and their families. This approach allows NPs to intervene on broad issues affecting a client's quality of life, take a preventive approach to offset any potential threats to well-being, and identify trends within the community associated with recurring problems presenting in their practice. To appreciate the nature of the NP practice, apart from outlining role responsibilities, one needs to further gain an appreciation for the challenges of role development, diversity among NP roles, and significance of expanded roles to professional growth.

Challenges of Role Development

Scope of practice can be viewed as a set of skills and a body of knowledge encapsulated within a boundary that is determined by legal and professional restraints. An expanded role can then be viewed as the grey or blurred area of practice extending beyond the accepted boundary of nursing but within a scope in which nurses are competent to provide care. In the beginning stages of role development, it is this grey area of practice in which practitioners struggle to determine if new skills and knowledge are congruent with the philosophical beliefs and standards of the profession. Further, the practitioner must gain recognition as a capable provider for newly selected aspects of care, and must determine the legal and professional implications of exploring new territory. During this period, NPs will move from novice to expert as they become efficient at performing new skills and integrating new knowledge into a nursing perspective. Simply stated, it is an area of practice in which there is intense activity to redefine the boundaries of nursing.

As these practitioners continue to define their new responsibilities, the ambiguity and confusion that is associated with the initial stages of role expansion will eventually clear. NPs must reflect on the balance between taking on new responsibilities and possibly giving up old ones while maintaining a nursing perspective. However, the process of role definition is never complete since the changing health care system is continually presenting new opportunities and challenges. For NPs, role development involves a continual re-evaluation of the nature of nursing as nurses search and conceptualize a broader dimension of practice.

With role definition comes new challenges such as reimbursement mechanisms, educational preparation, acceptance by consumers and other health professionals, legislation to support new role responsibilities, strategies for certification and continuing education, and the establishment of national and provincial professional associations. Without sufficient political, professional, educational and legal support, practitioners will continue to practice in limbo, facing the uncertainties of appropriate practice boundaries, and the risk of legal prosecution. As discussed in the previous chapter, certain factors play a significant role in creating the appropriate environment for change; however, the real motivation must come from within the profession itself, as nurses come together to redefine their roles and responsibilities in a changing health care system. The personal and professional rewards that are gained by such endeavors will alter the image of nursing for future generations to come.

Diversity Among Nurse Practitioners' Roles

Several factors influence the ability of NPs to develop roles in different settings: educational preparation, health care demands of the population served, availability of other health professionals to meet these demands, impact of health professionals on role development, support and guidance of individuals in power positions such as physicians and administrators, and professional and agency approval for expanded role activities. It is these factors which influence role development by creating a need for or emphasis on certain role functions. For example, a NP may have provided bereavement counselling in her last position. However, the social workers in her new employment presently provide this service. The NP may then provide other counselling services or negotiate with the social worker for sharing the responsibility. In order to be successful in implementing the role in different settings, practitioners have to respond to these external influences and make the appropriate adjustments in their roles. It is for these reasons that similarities and differences in role responsibilities among and between NPs in specialties exist.

This diversity can be interpreted as confusing and detrimental to the profession. However, it can be argued that each setting and specialty brings unique challenges. In order to be effective, the NP is required to remain flexible and sculpt a role congruent with nursing, and the needs of the setting and specialty.

It is the flexibility of the NP model that has made it desirable and successful in the dynamic health care system for such a long time. "The diversity among the role functions and skills is not a negative aspect of advanced practice. It simply demonstrated the multiplicity of opportunities available for nurse functioning at this level."[3] Although certain broad standards need to be set in order to protect the public, there should always be flexibility in the regulation of the role to allow for creative and professional reflection.

Role Responsibilities

The blending of knowledge and skills of nursing and selected aspects of medicine allows NPs to examine the complexities of the client's experience from a more holistic perspective. In the illness experience, it is not only the treatment of the disease that can be a priority to the client but the many interrelated health issues created or intensified by its presence. Although diagnosis and management of illness is considered part of their role, NPs have the ability to identify and intervene on the issues created by the impact of illness and to promote positive changes through healthy behaviours. "NPs possess the skills and knowledge to make a significant contribution to the maintenance of health through their defined role in the management of illness and the promotion of health."[4]

Although the main focus of the NP's role is clinical practice, it is possible to include other activities such as education, consultation and research as other aspects of the role. (Table 1) Traditionally, NPs have been employed in primary settings. However, there are nurses who are performing expanded role functions in tertiary care settings. These nurses are called nurse practitioners, expanded role nurses, and clinical nurse specialist/nurse practitioners, to name a few.[5] Although the differences in titles have created confusion for both the employer and the consumer, some of these nurses have developed a role in their specialties around expanded activities and the subroles associated with the clinical nurse specialist.[6,7] The role of the NP in secondary and tertiary care settings has not been studied as extensively as the role in primary care. Whether these titles, including NP, will be used to describe roles in tertiary care settings in the future or merged under the umbrella of one common title has yet to be determined.

NPs must have not only extensive knowledge to intervene appropriately in the many types of potential clinical situations, but the skills and qualities essential to be a successful role developer. They must be risk-takers, possess an ability to envision all the potential possibilities for nursing practice and role development, have inquiring minds, remain flexible, articulate clearly, and demonstrate leadership skills.[3,8,9,10] As role developers, they are required to identify and develop a nursing perspective in new areas of health care, utilize and conduct research to guide practice, articulate and disseminate knowledge to other nurses and members of the health care team and assist others in their practice.[3,8] To remain competent in their practice, they must be committed to lifelong learning.

Nurse practitioners are capable of independent (without the approval of the physician) and collaborative problem-solving and decision-making. Although the word 'independent' has been the crux of disagreement between nursing and medicine in Ontario, the then president of the College of Nurses emphasized the importance of collaborative relationships, autonomy in decision-making and accountability for nursing practices.[11] In addition, the Nurse Practitioners' Association of Ontario released a statement on independent practice. They stated:

> Nurse Practitioners, who meet educational and practice requirements and who register in the proposed Extended Nursing Practice Level of the College of Nurses of Ontario, will have the authority to make independent judgements regarding a client's health status and use of appropriate diagnostic tests and treatment plans that may include prescriptive drugs. They will also have the authority to communicate a diagnose to the client.[12]

The Association endorsed the Ministry of Health's decision to employ NPs in primary health care settings, working in collegial relationships with other members of the multidisciplinary team. In addition, they acknowledged the potential for nurse-initiated health care projects that may not require the employment of medical staff. The issue of independent nurse practice is far from being resolved in Ontario. The major tasks that face nursing in the future are to come to grips with whether independent practice is appropriate for the profession, and if yes, what strategies will be required to address the legal and professional issues emanating from such a move.

Table 1

Role Functions of Nurse Practitioners Clinical Practice

Clinical Practice	• Provides care to clients independently or collaboratively in primary, secondary or tertiary care settings, and outreach programs. • Assesses the needs of clients by collecting, integrating, and validating a wide range of complex information from various sources. • Collects a comprehensive health data base through a history and physical examination. • Diagnoses illness and health-related issues according to legal, professional, and institutional criteria. • Prescribes medication according to legal, professional, and institutional criteria. • Orders tests according to legal, professional, and institutional criteria. • Performs nursing and selected medical interventions depending on the setting and according to legal, professional, and institutional criteria. • Evaluates outcomes of patient care. • Documents findings and plan of care. • Acts as a patient/family advocate. • Promotes continuity of care through continued assessment and evaluation of patient care. • Provides counselling and health teaching on a variety of illnesses and health-related issues. • Communicates and collaborates with the multidisciplinary team, patient, and family in setting mutual goals.
Leadership in Clinical Practice	• Participates in the development of scientifically based clinical standards, policies, and procedures. • Identifies barriers to providing quality of patient care. • Acts as a resource to nurses. • Demonstrates leadership skills and expertise consistent with advanced nursing practice. • Demonstrates skill in role development.
Education	• Contributes to the dissemination of nursing knowledge. • Participates in the development of community programs. • Participates in the development of educational programs for health care providers, clients, and families. • Maintains competency of practice through the use of resources and educational programs.
Consultation	• Accepts and makes referrals to other health care professionals. • Consults with other members of the health care team. • Represents nursing on internal/external committees for political initiatives and matters affecting nursing clinical practice.
Research	• Critically analyses and demonstrates research-based practice. • Initiates and conducts nursing and collaborative research. • Disseminates research findings.

Importance of Expanded Practice to the Nursing Profession

From a professional prospective, expanded practice involves a process of role development in which nurses explore new opportunities and redefine the scope of nursing practice. It is a necessary process for maintaining the relevance of nursing's contribution to a dynamic health care system and, to a large extent, is the impetus for growth within the profession.

The change in the nature of nursing that results from the activities of practitioners such as CNSs and NPs, as well as the way nursing is viewed by the public and other health professionals, can be perceived as a potential risk or benefit depending on one's perspective. Although it is always difficult to predict the effect of role expansion on the profession as a whole, it is probable that these responsibilities or selected aspects of them will be incorporated into general nursing. The acceptance of physical assessment into nursing practice is an example of how a new skill performed by NPs eventually influenced the education and practice of nurses in general.[13] "Through their ability to develop a nursing role in a new area of health care and to disseminate the knowledge to other nurses, nurse practitioners changed the focus of nursing practice towards holistic assessment."[13] Regardless of whether the expanded role activities of practitioners are accepted within the scope of nursing practice, the way nurses view their profession and contribution will be altered. The question then remains how our experiences with role expansion today will affect nursing's growth and relevancy in the future health care system.

Chapter Three

Carving a Role...

Shari Glenn, Dorothy Anne Mills, Bob Harris, Deb Bisnaire, Janet Pinelli, Barbara Love, Anna Giallonardo, Rita Schreiber, Chris Patterson

In Canada, NPs have participated in the development of roles in community health centres, health service organizations, northern medical clinics, northern nursing stations, occupational and acute care settings. Although the idea of other types of employment arrangements, such as independent practice, has been discussed, most NPs are hired as employees of a particular agency. In this chapter, the personal accounts of NPs working in primary health care and acute care settings are outlined. Professional, legal and clinical issues of role development will be discussed for various practices.

Techniques for role development are as essential for success to NPs as their clinical skills. The survival of the NP initiative will depend on the ability of NPs to carve a role congruent with the demands of the health care system. A new NP can be led to believe that developing a role is straightforward, but in reality it requires planned strategies skillfully executed. Without proper planning, successful implementation of the role can be jeopardized by the practitioner's inability to recognize and deal with the many issues which can arise. From the perspectives of NPs in different settings and specialty areas, you will gain further insight into the complexities of an expanded practice.

... In a Family Practice in a Rural Community Health Centre...

Shari Glenn

Uniqueness of Rural Settings

The practice examples and comments provided are my own personal experiences and opinions accrued over a ten-year practice history in rural Newfoundland and Ontario. Defining the term 'rural' is unfortunately not straightforward. Presently, there is no universally accepted definition of this term. For many urban dwellers, 'rural' means "anything that is smaller than here and is probably inhabited by cows." There are, however, two important characteristics presented repeatedly in a variety of definitions: low population density and a unique diversity for each rural area.[1]

The practice of rural nursing is within the physical and sociocultural context of these unique settings.[2] Long and Weinert proposed a rural nursing theory consisting of six key concepts: isolation, distance, self-reliance, lack of anonymity, insider/outsider, and old-timer/newcomer perspectives.[3] These concepts are present in all rural settings to some degree and can influence the NP's role.

Currently, I practice in a rural setting approximately 1100 square kilometers in size, with a population unevenly distributed across six municipalities. Communities vary in size from 25 to 800 individuals, with seniors and children comprising the largest proportion. Twenty percent of the adult population has less than Grade 9 education, with 50% to 60% not having received high school certificates. Families generally have a lower income than those reported in the county, with general welfare assistance doubling in the winter months. One half of the population works in occupations with little job security and a high risk of injury.

The majority of seniors live in the most isolated areas of the region, making delivery of care to these individuals difficult.

Although independence, dignity, self-sufficiency, and hardiness are valued characteristics of older adults, these traits (in combination with limited resources) can contribute to delay in seeking health care until the rural elder is quite ill.[4] For example, I was conducting a clinic held once a week in a satellite village, accommodating residents unable to travel to the central facility located 60 miles away. During a busy afternoon, a client asked if I would come with him to visit a neighbour. There had been a snowstorm the day before; today, there was no smoke coming out of the chimney. We found him collapsed on the floor, cold, dehydrated, and in some respiratory distress. With the help of several neighbours, we positioned him securely on a stretcher with his oxygen and intravenous bags. Three weeks later, the gentleman returned for follow-up care. He stated that he had considered coming for a check-up before his collapse but did not want to bother anyone for just a cold. The self-reliance of residents makes education for early detection and prevention of illness important. In addition, education on the appropriate use of health care resources and providers is an ongoing challenge. Multiple approaches can be used to reach the rural population, such as articles in the local paper, speaking at senior luncheons or women's institute meetings, presenting displays at fall fairs, attending children's play groups, and generally being visible and accessible.

The unique nature of settings and the values and beliefs of the residents influence an NP's practice and the manner in which health care services are provided. The NP is a community-based provider who incorporates into practice the broader concepts of primary health care: comprehensiveness, accessibility, continuity, family-centred, and self-actualizing care.[5] In order to provide health services congruent with the needs of residents and their community, the NP must assess and respond to a variety of health and illness issues. For example, when I worked in an outpost in the Northwest Territories, the majority of time was spent in a curative role because of the community needs and the scarcity of resources. During my urban experience, clinical activities involved educating and counselling clients. Again my role functions in this setting were dictated by the presence of multiple resources and support from other providers. In a rural practice, I have used the knowledge of my past experiences and skills to develop a role that reflects a broader scope of nursing practice. However, unlike outpost nursing where the expanded nursing role is the norm, the NP's practice was new to this area, and people required education about the role through practical demonstration of my skills.

The specific health needs of the residents are probably no different from urban settings, but the strategies used to satisfy those needs are different. For example, attendance at parent support groups is complicated by transportation difficulties. Community culture also influences care delivery: an NP practising in the North would probably not plan a major health initiative in the spring of the year when the majority of residents are away camping. In a rural area, practitioners need to consider busy time periods, such as hunting seasons, harvest times, and hockey playoffs. Different activities within the community will vary among regions and within communities, and are important considerations when planning programs. Therefore, because of the differences in rural living compared to urban settings, it may be inappropriate to transplant urban policies and expectations to rural settings.

The Independent and Collaborative Role of the NP

Multidisciplinary health care teams are one way to deliver quality care in complex settings. The team providing service for this rural region is composed of a NP, primary health care nurse, two family physicians, and a health promoter, as well as professionals from nutrition, physiotherapy, chiropody, psychiatry, and social work. Although team members practise independently within their scope of practice, they can collaborate to provide a holistic approach toward the individual, family, and community. Team members are not required to obtain the physician's approval for care within their scope of practice. When differences of opinion arise, the professional with the greatest degree of competence in the area has the authority to make the final decision.[6]

The NP is capable of providing care independently across the health-illness continuum with the client and family. When appropriate, the NP works in collaboration with other members of the health care team at the centre or from collateral agencies. Emphasis is placed on holistic care, health promotion, and disease prevention. The most rewarding aspect of the role is the continuity in care offered to clients. The NP may offer preconceptual counselling to a young couple, and then later, be involved in their prenatal and postnatal care. As the child grows, the NP will perform well child examinations and anticipatory guidance for those colicky evenings. For the chronically ill patient, fostering health promoting and disease preventing behaviours, identifying and treating select acute episodes, monitoring for complications, and providing psychosocial support for the individual and family are part of the daily care provided by the NP.

In certain circumstances, the complexity of patient care makes it difficult for any one professional group to claim success in providing total care. It is only through a collaborative effort that the diverse issues of a client can be addressed. For example, isolation for clients is problematic in accessing health care services, especially in an emergency. A woman in crisis, living several kilometers from the closest neighbour or village, sought help from the NP. The only means of transportation, the family car, was not available because her husband used it for work. She was at home with two young children. She called the clinic, expressing uncontrollable feelings.

Obviously, management of the initial crisis is the first priority, but more importantly, long-term management and relationships need to be developed. Because of the potential safety issue, a child protection agency had to be notified. With the collaboration of the client, the agency would assess not only safety issues, but explore areas for assistance in tenuous family dynamics. Maintaining a therapeutic environment and a trusting relationship with the woman during this necessary yet stressful referral were of utmost importance. After the well-being of the children was confirmed, family meetings were arranged with the councillor, as well as home visits by the NP. In addition, following a health assessment, an endocrine imbalance was found, which prompted a medical referral. As the various problems were addressed, the woman began to feel more in control of her life, and had the courage and strength to address other issues. The transportation problem was partly resolved by utilizing the school bus system and enlisting a volunteer driver.

Many of the patient care issues in this example are long term, requiring the involvement of several professional groups. As an advocate of a client, the NP maintained a safe and secure environment, enabling clients to feel comfortable seeking assistance. Since NPs have a broad and in-depth knowledge base in nursing, they are capable of addressing various situations, taking into consideration the environment and culture of their clients. In addition, they have refined assessment skills which allow them to identify pertinent issues.

Collaborative practice is also important in prenatal care. The geographical area presents challenges to prenatal women. Clients are situated between two major centres offering midwifery services. However, because of the distance, midwives are not available for home births. As well, in order to access this service, women require transportation to drive the long distance to appointments in a variety of seasonal road conditions. Families who choose obstetrician care are faced with the same challenges. The situation is further complicated by the fact that few family physicians in the area practise obstetrics.

Shared-care arrangements have developed to minimize the problems in accessing health services. A schedule of visits, the role of the different caregivers, and a plan in case of an emergency are discussed among the NP, delivering caregiver, and client. The essential element of shared care is open communication among caregivers and client. Without good communication, the arrangement deteriorates, jeopardizing patient care.

In the prenatal process, the NP will provide a variety of services. Once the initial health assessment and the appropriate investigations are completed, education emphasizing health promoting behaviours for both client and baby becomes an important aspect of care. Normal healthy pregnancy and the early detection of prenatal problems are within the NP's scope of practice. If abnormalities are present, the appropriate caregiver is consulted. In addition, the involvement of the public health nurse, community social worker, nutritionist, health promoter, or physiotherapist may be indicated in the client's care.

Effective collaboration is dependent on professionals practising to the full extent of their respective expertise and bringing that expertise to the group in a co-operative manner. Flexible access to multiple resources is important in this setting since many clients have reported feeling uncomfortable in more formalized classes, and marginalized by their experiences in larger institutions.

In addition, the NP participates in ongoing community assessment. Broader community issues generally cannot be addressed in clinic visits or outreach sessions. There are many social and economic issues resulting in children arriving at school without lunch or breakfast, a significant number of depressed and suicidal teenagers, and adults who are no longer included in the unemployment statistics because they have given up on themselves and others. The NP has a responsibility to identify the socio-economic trends which compromise health and to assist the community to plan appropriate strategies to minimize their effects.

Barriers to the NP Role

The rural environment does present some challenges. Isolation and distance refer not only to geography but to professional issues. The practitioner experiences isolation from professional peers, resources, and continuing education programs.[7,8] Being the sole NP in a community can at times be a professionally lonely experience. As rewarding as being part of a multidisciplinary team can be, there are times when one seeks the perspective of another NP. Contracting with a health science library to provide literature searches and current awareness packages is an innovative solution which addresses the lack of local resources. As well, availability of continuing education through distance programs is essential for remaining competent.

Lack of information about the nature of the role and contributions of NPs to health care are major barriers. Individuals who have worked with NPs either as colleagues or clients are aware of the appropriateness of the role. NPs have established their ability to provide high quality care.[9] However, it is not enough to demonstrate on the basis of individual relationships the merits of the role. NPs must seek out opportunities to describe the role through publications, conference presentations, meetings with local members of parliament, and by never refusing an opportunity to speak about their contributions.

Regardless of how much support is gathered for NPs, without legislation the role will never be legitimized. Presently, for most of Canada, prescribing, diagnosing, and laboratory and radiological investigations are performed under protocols developed by the physician and NP. If the situation is not addressed within a protocol, the NP must obtain an order or refer to the physician. Protocols vary among organizations, with their development dependent on the individual personalities and policies of the institution. The lack of control and consistency in the NP's scope of practice compromise the integrity of the profession.

Legislation which protects special interest groups will limit the contributions of other competent practitioners and narrow the approach to client care.[10] When studying human health resource needs, one should not assume that roles of key personnel, such as physicians and nurses, will continue to follow the same patterns as in the past.[9] The system must change not only to reflect economic circumstance, but more importantly, move from an illness-driven system to one that values health and empowers people.

The rural community will continue to be an ideal setting for the NP. NPs offer a unique blend of skills and attributes to clients and the team, such as clinical skills, adaptability and flexibility, assessment skills, organization, independence, self-confidence, emergency skills, education, and public relation skills.[11] Lassiter proposed that rural nursing demands from practitioners appropriate attitudes and a wide range of knowledge and skills beyond basic education.[12] Being a rural NP is a challenging and unique experience. The setting requires a great deal of knowledge and skill from practitioners, but also allows for the autonomy and creativity to practice nursing as it was meant to be.

... In a Family Practice Unit Affiliated with a University Teaching Hospital...

Dorothy-Anne Mills

In the late 1970s, a family practice unit opened at McMaster Medical Centre in Hamilton. Three nurses who had recently graduated with a baccalaureate degree in nursing science, two family physicians and a family physician-who was also a paediatrician-were the initial health professionals of the unit. Because nurses were determined to function in roles different from traditional office nurses, they enrolled and graduated from the first program for nurse practitioners at McMaster University. Through careful planning and collaboration by nurse practitioners and physicians, the unit gradually began to take shape and became known as the 'Family Practice Unit.' As a health service organization, clients registered with the unit can be seen by different health professionals, depending on their needs. Currently, there are six teams of nurse practitioners and family physicians providing care to approximately 7800 rostered clients. As a university teaching unit, there are expectations placed upon us. The major ones include:

1. *Service Objectives:* Provision of family-centred, coordinated and continuous care to a group of registered clients. This includes daytime as well as evening and weekend coverage.
2. *Educational Objectives:* Provision of an educational experience for medical doctors wanting to complete a two-year postgraduate training program in the specialty of Family Medicine.Provision of an educational experience for students in the Bachelor of Science in Nursing Programme.
3. *Scholarly Activities:* Participation in research activities as an investigator, co-investigator or participant, in addition to other scholarly activities such as writing papers.

The unit is organized so that a team physician is available for unit activities-the equivalent of three full days a week. At other times, he may be tutoring students in the undergraduate medical program or working on scholarly activities. When my physician is unavailable, there are always other staff physicians available to assist with problems and issues beyond my scope of practice.

For the past 25 years, I have had the pleasure of working with a family physician who is also a paediatrician. He has been a keen advocate and supporter of the role. Together, we provide services to 1,200 clients in our team, including many three- or four-generation families who have been with us for over 20 years. Attached to our team are three doctors enrolled in the Family Medicine Residency Program and a third year Bachelor of Science in Nursing student. The team's goals are to provide holistic quality care for clients and their families, taking into account their sociocultural, economic, and developmental status.

In clinical practice, NPs work in both independent and collaborative roles. I provide health care to individuals and families in the unit, in community settings, or on the telephone. NPs go out into the community either independently or with other team members to visit chronically ill clients who are physically or emotionally unable to attend the clinic, nursing home residents, and institutionalized clients. The types of services that I provide include:

(a) acute care for common episodic problems;
(b) chronic care management for stable problems;
(c) well person care, including well child and well adult visits with pap smears and immunization if required;
(d) advice and health instruction, such as obesity counselling and lifestyle changes;
(e) women's health care, including visits for family planning, vaginitis, breast problems, menstrual problems, prenatal, and postpartum visits;
(f) management of psychosocial issues, including anxiety, depression, adjustment reactions, and family problems;
(g) telephone calls to provide information about test results, medication changes, and screening clients' concerns to decide if a problem can be managed with telephone advice or by an appointment; and
(h) facilitation of community links for clients receiving services from community agencies.

Carving a role in the unit has been relatively problem free, partly because my physician believed that not all visits to the unit are illness-related. As a practising paediatrician in the community for a number of years, he identified little in his daily office routine that required his extensive knowledge and training. He viewed his clients from a holistic perspective, recognizing their role within their family and community. He also acknowledged his comfort level in dealing with the illness and curative model of health care, but not with the teaching, counselling, preventive, and palliative aspects of care.

Through ongoing dialogue with the physician, we discussed areas of similarities and differences in our roles. The physician has the depth and breadth of knowledge for analysing complex medical problems, while the NP has the knowledge and skill to initiate more health promotion and disease prevention strategies. There was also a large grey area where either the physician or NP is competent to provide care. Issues in the grey zone included, but were not limited to, treatment of uncomplicated acute illnesses such as earaches, frequency of urination, and upper respiratory tract infections.

Despite similarities in practice, our approach to patients can be different. For example, if a young female teenager comes with a form requiring a physical examination to participate in sports, in addition to the physical examination I would take the opportunity to discuss contraception, smoking, and alcohol. Health teaching would include information on the types of birth control available, possible side effects, benefits and risks associated with different methods of contraception, as well as ways she can protect herself against sexually transmitted diseases. As for the physician, he would complete the examination, answer questions, and sign the form. The opportunity to discuss contraception and other behaviours could be lost. Because of my nursing perspective, I try to assess and plan with the client strategies to promote healthy behaviours as part of every encounter.

The following examples demonstrate the independent and collaborative nature of the NP's role in the unit. A gentleman, generally in good health, was diagnosed with hypertension in 1994. His blood pressure was controlled with two medications. In a routine follow-up visit, I checked his blood pressure, weight and pulse, listened to his heart sounds, reviewed the treatment plan and his compliance with medications, discussed side effects, and reinforced the importance of a healthy lifestyle. In this case, I managed the patient independently because his condition was stable.

In contrast to the above scenario, clients with unstable or undiagnosed problems may be seen by the physician. For example, a frail, elderly client admitted not feeling well with a new medication. For this reason, she discontinued her medication after only two weeks. Two nights later, she 'blacked out' and fell backwards onto her bed. On my examination in the clinic, abnormal findings were found, and the physician was consulted. Together we reviewed and revised the plan of care. Before leaving, I reinforced the need for compliance with the medications, and the nature of the scheduled tests to determine the cause of her syncope. Generally, a physician is consulted when a client has a complex, undifferentiated, or unstable illness. Even though the physician will take on the responsibility of managing the illness, I will continue to remain involved by providing health teaching, support, and promoting healthy behaviours.

As an educator, I am recognized by the Department of Family Medicine and the School of Nursing for my contributions to both family medicine residents and nursing students. As an Associate Clinical Professor with the Department of Family Medicine and an Associate Member of the School of Nursing, I share with the physician the responsibility of monitoring the care provided by family practice residents and student nurses. Educational responsibilities include role-modeling an approach to care; assisting students and residents with interviewing techniques, history-taking, physical assessment skills and procedures; facilitating students' problem-solving abilities in providing care in the clinic, in the community, and during telephone calls; and providing feedback, as well as evaluating documentation of care. As a role model for health teaching, counselling, and preventative aspects of health care, family practice residents in particular are exposed to a broader dimension of health than the traditional illness/curative model of care.

In addition to providing educational opportunities to students, I participate in the unit's educational events such as obstetrical and paediatric rounds. From 1975 to 1983, I was a faculty member in the Nurse Practitioner Program. Since 1983, I have been a tutorial leader in a primary care and physical assessment course offered to nursing students. I am a founding member of the Family Practice Unit Education Committee. This is an important committee with the mandate to evaluate educational experiences in the unit and trouble-shoot where there are program, resident, or nursing student difficulties. I am also an active member of the Department of Family Medicine Appointments, Promotion and Tenure Committee, a committee that reviews all initial and continuing appointments for full- and part-time faculty members in Family Medicine. As charge nurse of the unit for many years, I was the nursing representative for the Family Practice Administrative Committee.

Although I am not as active in research at present, I have had the opportunity to be a principal investigator and co-investigator in several studies which have been published. I was a co-investigator for a large well baby study which received funding for three years.

Developing the Role of the NP

In my opinion, there is definitely a future for NPs in units/clinics associated with hospitals/institutions. Particularly where there are learners and university attachments, the environment provides NPs with opportunities to participate in clinical practice, education, research, and committees which can help shape how health care can be delivered. However despite the success story of NPs in the Family Practice Unit, there is a considerable amount of work that needs to be done to facilitate a more widespread acceptance of NPs in these settings. The following were identified as future considerations for maximizing the role of NPs:

1. Administrators and consumers must have a greater awareness of the capabilities of qualified NPs and their contributions to the health care system. Consumer education about the role of the NP could be accomplished through newspaper/magazine articles, radio, and television interviews.

2. Educational opportunities must be readily available to prepare registered nurses to competently perform expanded role functions in a specialty.
3. Reimbursement mechanisms and employment opportunities that allow NPs to utilize their knowledge and skills must be identified.
4. Closer alliance between NPs, physicians, and other health care providers with acceptance of each other's unique contributions to the health care system should be fostered in clinical settings and within educational programs.
5. Collaboration with educators and researchers in universities and colleges will assist NPs in developing the necessary skills for teaching, research, and other scholarly activities.

Despite the fact there has been a slow movement towards integrating NPs into these settings, their skills would make a difference in the way health care is delivered. From my perspective, NPs in the Family Practice Unit have contributed to the team approach of providing care in a more holistic manner.

.... In Orthopaedics....

Bob Harris

In a report entitled Expanded Role Nurse Project, Haddad reported that escalating health care costs and province-wide constraints caused provincial restriction of the number of physicians graduating in specialty areas.[13] Nurses with expanded knowledge and skills were proposed as al ternatives to residents. As part of the process for implementing expanded role nurses, Haddad conducted a survey in London, Ontario, to "identify the needs and concerns, as well as the strengths within University Hospital which are pertinent to, and will enhance or impede the appropriate utilization of Expanded Role Nurses."[13] Health professions in both medicine and nursing were interviewed for their insight into a more expanded role for the nurse and their perceptions of the demands' of clinical practice. The findings of this survey provided the incentive for the development of nurses in different specialties who were capable of meeting the increasing clinical demands, providing staff education, developing and using research, and establishing a communication link between physicians and nurses.

As part of the training for the role, nurses were required to be enroled in the Master's of Science in Nursing at the University of Western Ontario. An amended education program was established using the available educational opportunities within the Faculties of Medicine and Nursing, as well as in University Hospital. The curriculum included courses on nursing theory, as well as the clinical, educational, and research components of practice. In addition to the Master's program, courses within the medical school applicable to the areas of specialty were taken in anatomy, physiology, pathophysiology, and disease processes.[14] A professor at University Hospital was responsible for developing the expertise of the nurses in physical assessment.

In the beginning, there were expanded role nurses (ERNs) in Internal Medicine, Neurosurgery, Cardiology, Orthopaedics, and Cardiovascular Surgery. Presently, the University Campus of London Health Science Centre employs fifteen ERNs in the specialties of Neurosurgery, Neurology, Cardiology, Cardio-thoracic Surgery, Orthopaedics, Nephro-Urology/Dialysis, Palliative Care, Liver and Renal Transplant, and Arrhythmia service, with plans to introduce additional positions.

Of all the expanded role nurse positions at University Campus, orthopaedics was one of the first developed because of the number of patients admitted to the service, and the necessity for an advanced nurse practitioner to assist with the unique needs of a surgical area. Initially, the role involved working with one orthopaedic surgeon from the arthroplasty service. However, as the role evolved, I have acquired additional responsibilities with three other arthroplasty surgeons. My orthopaedic patients are primarily composed of 60- to 80-year-old patients who require or have had a total knee or hip joint replacement (arthroplasty). Although most patients tend to be elderly, there is a small percentage of adolescents and middle-aged individuals. There is also a smaller number of patients admitted for orthopaedic trauma or other conditions such as osteomyelitis, rheumatoid arthritis, or bone metastasises. Because it is a referral centre, patients are often composed of those requiring more complicated surgery or those with a higher surgical risk due to pre-existing medical problems.

For some time, my position as an advanced practitioner in orthopaedics was the only one in the city. However, Victoria Campus created a similar position. The Clinical Nurse Specialist/Nurse Practitioner (CNS/NP) at Victoria Campus works primarily with a different orthopaedic population.

Roles and Responsiblities

As an ERN, my role includes the subroles of clinical practice, research, education, and consultation. The role of a change agent, often attributed to the clinical nurse specialist, is part of the responsibilities of the ERN. In the early stages of role development, I spent most of my time in the inpatient area. Since then, the focus of my practice has shifted to the outpatient and preadmission clinics. Consultations for off-service clients throughout the hospital are also followed on a regular basis.

On the inpatient unit, I am responsible for the admission of patients and pre-operative teaching. The admission process includes obtaining a history and review of body systems, performing physical examinations and ordering routine diagnostic tests, treatments, medications, and consultations. A holistic approach to the history allows for the development of a comprehensive database which is used post-operatively for discharge planning and prevention of complications. I have the authority in the hospital to initiate certain diagnostic tests and treatments outlined in established protocols. Having privileges in ordering tests allows me the freedom to act efficiently on behalf of the patient, especially if physicians are not available. With respect to pre-operative teaching, it involves a wide variety of health-related issues for both patient and family, and includes a review and clarification of the surgery and treatment protocols.

In the post-operative period, I am involved with assessing complications, interpreting laboratory and diagnostic tests, monitoring the patient's response to the hospital experience, and determining their readiness for discharge. Ongoing follow-up has proven beneficial in early identification and treatment of problems. For example, a patient was admitted and treated for multiple injuries. Prior to the transfer, I reviewed the X-rays and identified a fractured wrist which had not previously been noted. The patient's wrist was casted, resulting in no adverse effect to the patient or liability to the hospital.

Communication with the patient, family, and members of the multidisciplinary team is a vital component of the role. With other members of the team, rationale for specific medical orders or treatment is shared. As a patient advocate, I ensure the patient's participation in decisions involving their care. I often spend time with the patient and family addressing and clarifying concerns. Because surgeons spend a great deal of time in surgery, they are not always available to talk with or answer questions of the patient and family. Making time to listen and bridging the gap in communication between doctor, patient, and family may be one of the most important functions of the role. In the case of an emergency, having access to consultants allows for more expedient care. In addition, responsibilities for communicating patient progress extend into the community. Transfers to home hospitals are coordinated by contacting family physicians, referring to community support systems, and dictating discharge summaries.

In the outpatient clinic, I primarily follow patients who have undergone total joint replacement surgery. During the visit, I will assess the function of the joint, discuss pain control, address all the patient's concerns, including non-orthopaedic problems, and discuss the results of radiographs. If abnormalities are detected beyond my scope of practice, or the patient requests to see the physician, the consultant will be notified. In complex situations, I will collaborate with the consultant on the treatment plan.

As well, I may assess a new referral for surgery in the clinic. In this situation, the history is focused on the chief complaint as compared to an overall screening history and physical examination done on admission or in the preadmission clinic. After discussing my findings, the consultant will see the patient, make a diagnosis, and discuss the risks and benefits of surgery. As before, I will answer any questions or clarify information. Educational pamphlets and a quick review of the surgery may be given to the patient. Specific diagnostic tests required for the preadmission clinic will be ordered by either the ERN or consultant on a standard preadmission form.

The orthopaedic service started to do preadmission histories and examinations in 1990. I was involved with the development of this initiative, and at the time performed about 50 assessments per year. In 1994, the preadmission clinic opened, increasing the number of patients seen by me to over 225 patients per year. In 1996, the number of patients seen in the clinic increased to 350. Because the preadmission clinic is a priority of the hospital, I remain flexible to accommodate the needs of the clinic and clients. I replace residents unable to attend clinic, and act as a liaison between the clinic and other patient care areas.

During assessment, the purpose is to obtain a comprehensive overview of the patient's health status. The history includes assessment of active and inactive health problems, review of body systems, risk factors for surgery, family history and social information (especially regarding home management after surgery), discharge plans, and the patient's ability to get to physiotherapy . The physical examination includes a general overview of all body systems and an in-depth musculo-skeletal assessment. Other specialized tests may be preformed depending upon the patient's situation. The comprehensive review often results in identification of additional or potential problems in the perioperative period.

It is the responsibility of the ERN to write the appropriate orders based on the findings of the history and physical examination. If abnormal findings are found, they are reviewed either with the Internal Medicine physician or consultant. Preoperative teaching and clarification of issues around surgery are discussed, and any questions answered to promote informed consent. Discharge planning may be initiated by the ERN or the preadmission nurse.

Being involved in the three clinical areas has provided unique opportunities for following the patient through the hospital experience, and identifying the strengths and weaknesses of the system influencing patients' recovery. Major contributions to patient care have occurred because of the continuity of care and communication among units. For example, in the past, patients received a narcotic and muscle relaxant in the inpatient unit prior to the residents attempting to relocate dislocated hips. During rounds, an anaesthetist brought to our attention the danger of this practice without the benefit of readily available resuscitation equipment and staff to monitor the patient after the procedure. After receiving this information, I was successful, with administrative support, in having the location of these procedures changed.

Researcher Role

I am a member of the Nursing Research Committee and previously was involved in the examination of a research utilization model for the Nursing Division. While in the Master's program, I completed a study on the nurse's use of the Morse Fall Scale. As a key member of an injury prevention group, we have implemented and evaluated the use of the Morse Fall Scale to reduce patient falls throughout the hospital. Collaborative research initiatives have included evaluating a drainage reinfusion system for arthroplasty patients and various other orthopaedic studies primarily involving patients who have undergone joint replacements. Research findings affecting orthopaedic nursing practice are shared with the nursing community. As well, I have acted as a resource for nurses and students in the unit in identifying research ideas and activities. Future nursing and collaborative research projects to evaluate newly developed clinical pathways for joint replacement are planned with the ERN taking a leadership role.

Educator Role

In addition to frequent informal teaching, I have conducted numerous inservices and presented at Nursing Rounds, as well as at local and national conferences of the Canadian Orthopaedic Nurses Association (CONA). Yearly musculoskeletal assessment and care of the orthopaedic patient workshops are given to nursing students at the University of Western Ontario. As a preceptor, observational experiences are provided for university, college, and high school students. As program chair for continuing education of the local CONA chapter, I organized four to five continuing education sessions per year for orthopaedic nurses. I am currently the national chairperson for Continuing Education with the Canadian Orthopaedic Nurses Association.

Consultant and Change Agent

Throughout the years, I have been a member of many hospital and nursing committees including Nursing Research, Quality of Worklife, Collaborative Practice, Falls Task Force, Morse Fall Scale Implementation and Evaluation Committee, Orthopaedic Interdisciplinary Working Group (developing clinical pathways), and the Musculo-skeletal and Rehabilitation Services Accreditation team. As a consultant, I act as a resource to providers on the orthopaedic unit, physicians secretaries, and other staff in different departments of the hospital. I collaborate with the inpatient unit coordinator and managers, discussing the needs of clients and staff, as well as being available to other orthopaedic centres. I have been involved in developing standards of care for new equipment, such as drainage reinfusion systems, for arthroplasty patients.

Challenges in Role Development

Nursing educators and other nurses have challenged the creation of a nursing position which they perceived as a 'physician assistant.' However, this perception is changing as the nurse practitioner role receives more public and political attention. The role of the ERN in orthopaedics is more than a resident replacement or physician assistant. The ERN is an advanced nurse practitioner and functions from a nursing perspective. Many of the role responsibilities are similar to the subroles of the clinical nurse specialist. The expanded role functions, such as diagnosing and prescribing, are similar to those described in Ontario for the generalist nurse practitioner.

When I first began in the role, physicians challenged the need for master's preparation. However, in order to fulfil role expectations, this level of preparation is required. A higher level of education prepares practitioners for the advanced level of judgment required in the role. In addition, NPs must have a strong 'nursing identity' if the role is to be rooted in nursing. One can easily become consumed by the physician's needs. Administrative support, which values the involvement of the ERN in nursing education and research, is important for maintaining a balanced perspective. A dual reporting structure is probably the best arrangement because it balances the demands and expectations of both medicine and nursing.

Challenges in role development have been related to multiple changes in the job description and reporting structure as a result of restructuring. Role overload and attempting to meet everyone's expectations has resulted in long hours. Compensation has only recently been addressed and now more accurately reflects the responsibility and long hours.

Several strategies have been used to relieve role stress. Initially, a project coordinator met with the ERNs to discuss issues, mediate problems, and support the ERNs through the process of role development. Eventually, a manager assumed the responsibilities of the project coordinator. Group meetings of all the ERNs were held regularly to discuss issues and strategies for overcoming barriers and to provide support to one another. The development of medical directives has been beneficial for outlining acceptable boundaries to expanded role activities. In addition, there has been flexibility from administration and physicians for the ERN to participate in professional development activities and continuing education activities, as well as in scheduling time off.

The current health care system does not recognize the advanced skills and autonomous decision-making required for the acute care role. Without legislation to support the expanded role functions, there is fear among advanced nurse practitioners of liability and difficulty maintaining efficient care. Currently, discussions with patients must be guarded to avoid any type of medical diagnosis, risks of surgery, and prognoses. Censored communication of this type can disadvantage clients seeking clarification or information about their care.

In spite of these problems, the ERN's role has broadened the scope of nursing and created opportunities for nurses to stay at the bedside. Exploring new avenues for nursing practice has been a rewarding challenge and essential for the growth of the profession. Adhering to one traditional perspective of how nursing practice should be enacted will only limit the profession and deny opportunity in the future.

...In Neurosurgery...

Deb Bisnaire

Despite the paucity of educational programs, and failure to resolve regulating issues, the NP is a valuable member of the tertiary care team. Known by a variety of titles, including Clinical Nurse Specialist/Nurse Practitioner (CNS/NP), Expanded Role Nurse (ERN) or Nurse Clinician, these nurses assume roles that combine expert nursing practice, traditional house officer responsibilities, and the coordinating skills of the case manager. At University Campus of London Health Science Centre in Ontario, in the division of neurosurgery, my experience with the expanded role nurse extends back to 1984. Proposed originally by medical staff in anticipation of resident shortages and hence a decreased ability to provide service to patients, the ERN's role evolved to meet patient care needs.

The Challenges of Role Evolution

Graduate educational programs are prerequisites to leadership in research and outcome-based practice. In addition to this formal preparation, the clinical setting will shape the evolution of each role. As outlined in Benner's work, the ERN evolves from novice to expert practitioner.[15] At each point along the continuum of role development, challenges will vary with the practitioner's circumstances and necessitate well-planned strategies. It seems reasonable to consider the process of role evolution in the clinical setting as a series of steps, and to outline some of the strategies which may be effective in overcoming barriers to role development.

I believe experienced nurses who are developing an expanded role face three main challenges. They must (a) narrow the gaps in their medical knowledge, skill, and judgment, (b) establish a collaborative relationship with the primary physicians and other key personnel, and (c) broaden and develop a unique nursing knowledge base.

Beginning ERNs will be overwhelmed by knowledge deficits. Regardless of the formal preparation, each clinical specialty will present unique challenges. The ability to take a history and perform a physical exam must be broadened from the nursing perspective to achieve medical diagnoses and plan care. For example, the neurosurgical ERN must be able to screen for potential medical or surgical problems, localize the area of the nervous system involved, and draft a diagnosis. In addition, ordering and interpreting diagnostic tests and prescribing pharmacologic and other therapeutic regimens require additional knowledge, skill, and judgment.

Strategies to meet these learning needs will vary but can include a one-to-one relationship with the physicians. The nurse and physician should practice together with minimal time and pressure constraints to review, discuss, and formulate plans of care for patients. Mentoring, role-modeling, and immediacy of feedback are invaluable in bridging the knowledge gap and in forging the relationship required for collaborative practice. In addition, formal educational opportunities must be sought and accessed. Resident and nursing teaching rounds, radiology review sessions, and courses offered at the nearest medical and nursing school may be available. Independent pursuit of information will be required and external connections with librarians, professional associations, and colleagues must be cultivated.

The second challenge for the novice practitioner is to establish collaborative relationships with the primary physician and other key players. Again, protected joint practice time is essential. Development of co-operation and mutual respect promotes appropriate use of providers and capitalizes on the strengths of the different professions.

The third task for novice ERNs is to develop their knowledge and expertise in nursing. For example, if one comes with expertise in the nursing management of patients with end stage renal disease, he/she must participate in initiatives to formulate care plans, act as consultant for the complex patient, and lecture and publish on nursing management. In this phase of role development, when practitioners are incorporating new knowledge into practice, there is a tendency to be overshadowed by anxiety over lack of expertise in the newly required knowledge and skills. By cultivating existing nursing expertise while developing the expanded role functions, the ultimate blending of the two perspectives into a holistic approach to care will occur.

With experience, the ERN becomes more skilled at clustering relevant findings from the history and physical examinations. Similarly, in investigation and treatment, the practice moves from diagnostic driven to more holistic and individualized plans of care. In short, the ERN moves from novice to experienced practitioner.

Challenges for the experienced ERN will include broadening medical expertise to include the management of health problems commonly associated with the specialty. For example, in surgical settings the management of medical problems such as coronary artery disease, diabetes mellitus, and chronic airway limitation is important to comprehensive care. The major challenge, however, at this point is to establish a clear sense of role identity. It will become apparent that the ability to diagnose/treat and recognize/manage complications is limited both from a legal and educational perspective. Within this traditional medical realm, the ERN's skills may be at the experienced practitioner level but will fall short of the clinical expert role achieved elsewhere. That is not to say that the ERN is incapable. Indeed if role satisfaction is achieved foremost through expanded role functions, a medical student is born. The key to successful resolution of this dilemma (and to longevity as an ERN) is to recognize and revel in the other components of the role that are at the expert level-the skill as a communicator, facilitator, and educator. This is the advanced nurse practitioner. With the addition of a much-broadened medical perspective, the ERN will excel in the independent aspects of the role and will continue to stretch the boundaries of nursing practice and expertise. It is the achievement of the blend that is unique to the ERN. Without this the ERN will become frustrated by limitations and mired in role confusion.

If the ERN can move from experienced to expert, he/she has found his/her niche, blending nursing with selected aspects of medical knowledge and skills to achieve excellence in patient care. As an advanced practitioner, the ERN continues to stretch the boundaries of nursing. Within the demands of patient care delivery, the ERN must find the time to pursue professional interests, such as clinical research, staff development, or patient teaching. Collaborators in practice and administrators must lend the support which enables longevity in practice.

Role Responsibilities in Neurosurgery

My current setting is in an academic health care centre. Neurosurgery accesses approximately 40 beds for patients admitted for investigation, surgery, and palliation. Inpatients may be critically or acutely ill and require general medical/ surgical care. There are four consultant neurosurgeons, two to three resident staff in various stages of training, and two full-time ERNs. Each ERN is affiliated with two consultants and, therefore, practises in a subspecialty (vascular versus epilepsy), as well as with the general neurosurgical population. All neurosurgical inpatients are thus 'attached to' a consultant, resident staff, and one ERN. In addition, each ERN spends one and a half days per week in outpatient clinics with the consultants, assessing both new and returning patients.

Inpatient nursing care for 60 patients (neurology, neurosurgery) is managed by two to three Nursing Coordinators (NCs) who coordinate, evaluate, and provide direct patient care. Nursing care is currently delivered in a model of total patient care by registered nurses (RNs), many of whom are baccalaureate prepared. Because staff nurses work 12-hour shifts and three shifts per week, much of the case management and discharge planning is facilitated by the NC. Changes in delivery of care, shorter length of stay, same-day admit procedures, and decreases in the number of middle managers involved in patient care necessitate changes in the role of the RN and other team members.

The patient care responsibilities in the inpatient area are shared among members of the team. Over time, the team evolves as its members evolve. Team members' loyalties and personal styles necessitate adjustments on a continuous basis. Although most team members' functions are interdependent, each player has dependent and independent components to his/her role. The variables that influence the roles assumed by different care providers include both educational and service components. Educational preparation and professional/legal limitations, time and day of the week, experience and skill, superseding responsibilities, and status of relationship with the individual patient or family will influence role responsibilities. The relative fluidity of role responsibilities necessitates excellence in communication among team members, mutual respect, and sensitivity to individual strengths and weaknesses.

For the ERN in neurosurgery, the prime responsibility is the patient. The ERN is expert and independent in identifying the patient's priorities, coordinating, communicating, and negotiating-a case manager. They are expert in assessment and interventions in nursing, and skilled and interdependent in the medical aspects of the role (may exceed a junior or less experienced resident). Interpreting clinical findings and establishing therapeutic relationships are at the expert level and a major responsibility; they are not, however, exclusive to the ERN. The ERN allows for greater efficiency (volume) and improved quality of care. Relative medical/nursing role responsibilities are summarized in Table 2.

Table 2

Relative Role Responsibilities - Medical and Nursing Tertiary Patient Care

Clinical Responsibility	Consultant	Resident	ERN	NC	RN
Admission history and physical	Occasional	✓✓	✓	--	Nursing Focus
Prescription pharmacology and other	✓	✓✓	✓✓	--	--
Invasive procedures	Occasional	✓✓	--	--	--
Surgery	✓✓	✓✓	--	--	--
Decision to admit, discharge, transfer	✓	✓	✓	input	input
Case Manager/ Coordinator	Occasional	✓	✓✓	✓	✓
Outpatient assessment/follow-ups	✓	Occasional	✓	--	--
Emergency Department assessment	Occasional	✓✓	✓	--	Nursing Focus
Communicate test results, etc.	✓	✓	✓✓	✓	✓
Initiate allied health referrals	✓	✓	✓✓	✓	✓

✓ minor responsibility
✓✓ major responsibility
-- no responsibility

In the outpatient department, the ERNs share responsibility with the consultant for assessing new referrals, post-operative, and follow-up patients. In collaboration with the physicians, they initiate treatment where indicated. The RN's availability in the outpatient area is very limited; therefore, it is the ERN who initiates teaching and arranges community support and health consultations.

The ERN also carries responsibilities for education (multidisciplinary team, patients, and family), consultation (internal and external to the hospital), and research. Educational offerings may be informal at the bedside or formal programs which vary from one hour to several days in length. All ERNs are members of the Nursing Research Committee whose aim is to promote research at the facility. Research has been both independent of and in collaboration with medicine. All ERNs are involved in dissemination of knowledge through presentations and publications.

Because the health care system is changing, the role of the ERN within the service is also changing. The NC shift to the administrative focus necessitates the RN to shift toward a case manager's role and the ERN to be more of an expert clinical resource. With movement to same-day admit procedures, adjustments in the responsibilities of the consultant, ERN, and resident will occur. For example, the responsibility of completing an admission history and physical examination will move from the resident, who obtained this information the night before surgery, to a different time and perhaps a different person. Similarly, as fewer specialty residents are trained and available for service, operating room and other technical assistance may be needed. As the primary role of patient care changes, adjustments in the ERN's secondary roles of education, research, and consultation will follow.

The Future of NPs in Tertiary Care

The NP role in tertiary care will continue to grow both in number and scope of practice. Nursing is prepared to push its traditional boundaries. Nurses are not only well educated but are practising longer than ever before. At the graduate level, clinical nursing has become an acceptable alternative to education and administrative career paths. Acute care facilities are looking to alternative models of providing care, and thus the more rigid professional boundaries are breaking down. Collaborative and interdisciplinary practice are the norm.

To be successful, the NP must be an excellent clinician who is satisfied by direct interaction with patients and families. The NP must be a skilled communicator with highly developed collaborative relationships with medical and nursing colleagues. He or she must be flexible-able to live with ambiguity, uncertainty, and ill-defined boundaries. Advanced practice necessitates constantly stretching the existing limits.[16] NPs must have a well-established sense of self-worth and must know the unique skills they possess. Support and respect from nursing, administration, and medical mentors are essential.[17]

...In Neonatal Intensive Care...

Janet Pinelli

Compared to the U.S., the role of the neonatal nurse practitioner (NNP) in Canada is relatively new. The first educational program to prepare advanced practice nurses in neonatal intensive care in Canada was established at McMaster University in Hamilton, Ontario, in 1986, as part of the Master of Health Science course of study. The graduates of this program have adopted the title, Clinical Nurse Specialist/ Neonatal Practitioner (CNS/NP) to describe their role.[18] The educational program was established following a provincial needs assessment,[19] determination of the acceptance of the role in Ontario, and the development of a role description.[18] This role has been evaluated extensively with respect to the effectiveness of the educational program,[20,21] effectiveness of the care provided by CNS/NPs,[22] and the impact of the role on the CNS/NP and other health care providers.[23]

Currently, the program at McMaster University is one of only two sites for formal NNP preparation in Canada, and the oldest. Plans are also underway to establish a program at Dalhousie University in Nova Scotia. Consequently, the largest number of CNS/NPs is in Ontario. The neonatal specialist component is currently available to students through the Clinical Health Sciences (Nursing) course of study at McMaster. As in the past, the component is also offered to post-master's students. The exact number of NNPs in Canada is unknown due to the lack of a national data base. The number of graduates from the McMaster program, who are working in the role in Canada, is 31. Therefore, based on informal sources, the number of formally prepared NNPs, who are working in the role in Canada, is probably less than 50.

The impetus for the introduction of the CNS/NP role in Ontario was a reduction in the number of paediatric residency positions and a change of focus in medical education.[19] "Reliance on physicians-in-training to provide all of the day-to-day care in a NICU on a 24 hour basis is no longer a viable option in many programs."[24] The CNS/NP role provides an opportunity for nurses to move beyond the basic level but continue in a clinical role. In the past, graduate education for nurses meant that they would move away from the bedside into management or academic positions.

In other NP specialties, the U.S. has taken the lead with regard to minimum educational requirements. However, the development of the role of the CNS/NP in Canada represents the cutting edge for the professional standard in neonatal critical care. The McMaster program combined the role of the CNS and NNP to prepare nurses at the graduate level to function as advanced practice nurses. The U.S. is moving toward graduate preparation as the minimum standard for NNPs, having started the role in the 1970s at the certificate level.[25] In a recent publication, the National Association of Neonatal Nurses (NANN) recommended graduate-level preparation for the NNP role by January 1, 2000.[26] This recommendation also included changes to the NNP certification eligibility requirements by that date to include successful completion of a graduate neonatal nursing educational program. The Canadian Nurses Association and the Canadian Special Interest Group of NANN also support graduate preparation for advanced practice roles in Canada.[27,28]

The role description of the CNS/NP reflects its combined nature: the role includes the components of direct clinical care, consultation, research, education, and administration.[18] Direct care comprises approximately 75% of the role, which is consistent with the NNP emphasis on clinical functions. However, 25% of the role of the CNS/NP involves non-clinical activities, which is not often the case for an NNP. An emphasis on non-clinical activities is congruent with the CNS aspects of the role.

The clinical component of the CNS/NP role involves direct care to neonates and their families. CNS/NPs provide initial and ongoing medical management of acute and chronic neonatal illnesses in consultation and collaboration with the neonatologist and other members of the interdisciplinary team. They order and perform a broad range of medical procedures in the diagnosis and treatment of neonates. Examples of the medical procedures performed by CNS/NPs include insertion and removal of chest tubes, umbilical and peripheral venous/ arterial catheters, endotracheal intubation, lumbar puncture, supra-pubic and ventricular reservoir taps, delivery room resuscitation and infant transport. In addition, CNS/NPs order medications, enteral and parenteral nutrition, blood and blood products, and ventilator adjustments, and order and interpret diagnostic and laboratory tests.

The clinical component also involves the provision of indirect care through consultation to staff on such issues as breast-feeding and developmental care. CNS/NPs communicate with parents regarding their infant's medical diagnosis, health status and prognosis, as well as results of clinical investigations. They assess parents' level of understanding, coping and support systems, and initiate necessary consultation with other health professionals. Finally, the CNS/NP collaborates with the interdisciplinary team, family, and referring physician in the infants' discharge planning and follow-up care.

CNS/NPs integrate the skills and knowledge from nursing and medicine within a broad framework of advanced nursing practice. To view the CNS/NP as merely a physician replacement or substitute, ignores the full potential of the role. In the acute phase of the neonate's illness, medical care is the appropriate focus for the CNS/NP. However, the impact of the advanced nursing aspects during this phase are manifested through such care priorities as pain management and the effect of environmental stimuli on the neonate. During the convalescent stage of the neonate's illness, the focus of medical care shifts to a greater emphasis on the advanced nursing aspects. Nutritional concerns and the impact of the disease on the infant's growth and development become the foci of care. Prevention of complications from the illness, as well as health promotion and disease prevention, are critical aspects of care that are the hallmark of advanced nursing practice. In addition, the daily involvement with families (from admission to discharge) provides opportunities for continuity of care that result in significant ongoing support for parents. The intense involvement with families also provides numerous opportunities for more general health promotion and health teaching.

The amount of time spent in different non-clinical activities varies with the individual CNS/NP and with the institution where they are employed. Educational activities represent a significant component for most CNS/NPs and include staff development, undergraduate and graduate nursing education, and outreach education. Staff development education involves formal and informal teaching, as well as the promotion of professional development and quality care through role modeling and collaborative care planning. CNS/NPs provide outreach education within their region and within the province.

Research and scholarly activities also comprise a large part of non-clinical activities. These activities include presentations at the provincial, national and international levels; publications; and acting as principal and co-investigators on funded and unfunded research projects. In addition, CNS/NPs facilitate nurses' understanding of the research process and utilization of research findings, and demonstrate the use of research findings as a basis for clinical decision making.

In addition to the NICU consultations mentioned previously, CNS/NPs respond to internal and external requests regarding the CNS/NP role or where the CNS/NPs unique expertise is required. These activities include task force and committee work, the development and revision of policies, procedures and protocols, and the critique of manuscripts and research grants. Consultation activities have been at the provincial, national, and international levels.

Due to the lack of nursing legislation related to the acute care role in Canada, CNS/NPs work under the authority of medical delegation. In Ontario, permission for CNS/NPs to perform the delegated medical acts predated the Regulated Health Professions Act and came from the Special Procedures Committee of the College of Physicians and Surgeons in 1985. This committee has representatives from the College of Nurses of Ontario, the Ontario Hospital Association, and the Registered Nurses Association of Ontario. The extensive research on this role, which was cited previously, supported the safety and efficacy of CNS/NPs in performing delegated medical acts. The only delegation issue which arose after the role was introduced was in relation to the co-signing of physicians' orders. The Public Hospitals Act prohibits non-physicians from signing medication orders, with the exception of dentists and veterinarians. The practice of co-signatures for all CNS/NPs orders quickly became a logistic impossibility for the neonatologists. Through a series of negotiations with the Special Procedures Committee and the various hospitals which employed CNS/NPs, the decision was made to allow the CNS/NPs to function under a broad medical directive with certain restrictions. Each hospital would then allow the CNS/NPs in their units to practice under the directive through the authority of the Medical Advisory Committee of each institution. The hiring institution would then be responsible for the certification and recertification of CNS/NPs to perform the delegated medical acts in accordance with hospital policies and procedures. The skills which are currently performed by CNS/NPs vary only slightly among the NICUs in Ontario. The medical directive gives the CNS/NP the authority to order and perform all procedures cited previously without a physician co-signature. The only restrictions in the directive are related to medications and certain blood products. The directive lists two groups of medications: those that can be ordered without a co-signature from a neonatologist, and those that require a co-signature prior to administration. The Medical Advisory Committee also gave the authority to update the lists through agreement among the chief neonatologist, pharmacist, and CNS/NPs.

Management rounds are conducted daily and the CNS/NP is part of the decision-making team. However, for the remainder of the time, the CNS/NPs function fairly autonomously, in that the amount of medical consultation is left to the individual's discretion. This autonomy is especially evident on evenings and nights, during transport, and in labour and delivery.

To date, the setting for NNPs in Canada has been limited to tertiary level units; however, the potential for employment settings is much more extensive. Opportunities for the introduction of NNPs into secondary-level units and follow-up clinics have been explored but have not come to fruition due to lack of funding for the proposed positions. Because of the broader master's preparation, NNPs can work in areas other than neonatal intensive care. As an example, two graduates of the McMaster program were clinical educators, and one was a hospital director of nursing. In addition, a number of the graduates have formal salaried appointments with educational institutions.

Challenges of Role Development

The success of the introduction of the NNP role in Ontario can be attributed to the well-planned strategies used by the multidisciplinary team at McMaster University. After the need for the role was identified and documented, the key stakeholders were involved in the development of the role activities and educational program. Most importantly, the role and program were systematically evaluated, and the results widely disseminated through publications and presentations. The introduction of the role in the NICU at McMaster University Medical Centre occurred with virtually no problems in terms of acceptance by administration. This was likely due to the fact that the directors of nursing and medicine were involved in the development of the role, as were the university counterparts in nursing and medicine. In the other hospitals, the first CNS/NPs to be employed in the NICU held a number of meetings with all levels of staff and involved every department that would come in contact with the CNS/NPs. Written information about the role and the research papers were also distributed to key stakeholders in the hospitals. The NICU administrative medical and nursing staff, and the staff nurses had also participated in the research surveys which preceded the role's introduction. In addition, the CNS/NPs were senior staff nurses in the units from which they came, and so were already well respected and supported. In this way, staff had knowledge of and a vested interest in the successful implementation of the role. The clinical and non-clinical role functions were well defined as a result of the aforementioned research; therefore, role ambiguity was almost non-existent.

In all hospitals which employ CNS/NPs, these advanced practice nurses are grouped with the other CNSs in their departments. They all participate in corporate activities and, as such, have been well integrated into the hospital system. The successful integration of the CNS/NP role into the larger hospital system, however, resulted in a degree of role conflict. This conflict relates to the limited time available to participate in non-clinical activities. Thus, the CNS/NP must restrict her participation in these activities to a greater extent than other CNSs who do not have as demanding a clinical component as the CNS/NPs. It is important for the CNS/NPs, therefore, to regularly communicate their role responsibilities as new staff come into the hospital system, in order to avoid misunderstanding and resentment. This communication is also important for non-nursing staff, many of whom have not worked with advanced nurse practitioners in an expanded role that includes a medical component. For the medical staff, the non-clinical activities need to be emphasized so that the magnitude of the role can be fully appreciated, and the differences between the medical and nursing aspects can be better understood.

The balance between clinical and non-clinical activities has remained the most difficult aspect of the CNS/NP role. Not surprisingly, financial implications exert the most powerful negative force in this delicate balance. CNS/NPs must remain competitive in terms of their cost to the system or risk replacement by less costly alternatives. CNS/NPs who devote 100% of their time to clinical activities would obviously be less expensive than those who spend 75% of their time clinically. However, the risk of professional burn-out and attrition would likely be much higher. In addition, the non-clinical activities are valued in the teaching hospitals where CNS/NPs are employed. For the time being, non-clinical activities appear to be protected from encroachment.

Another negative force in the balance of activities relates to the amount of shift work that is required in the role. Physician coverage in the NICU is a 24-hour per day, 365 days per year reality so that when CNS/NPs are substituted, the expectation is that shift work is a part of the clinical function. As more CNS/NPs replace physicians, there is an increasing burden of weekend, night, and holiday coverage. As stated previously, the NICU at McMaster University Medical Centre has the largest number of CNS/NPs in Canada. With 9.5 FTEs, this group provides clinical coverage that involves about 65% weekdays, and 35% weekends and nights. In a proposed expansion of the NICU, 15.75 FTEs will be needed, but the coverage will increase to 52% weekdays, and 48% weekends and nights. These numbers do not include holiday coverage, although there is currently at least one CNS/NP on the unit for every holiday. The expectation of shift work may deter some nurses from pursuing this career path, while others will accept the hours as long as financial remuneration remains competitive and the role is professionally satisfying.

There is no question, in terms of the medical component of the role, that overlap exists between the CNS/NP and the physician. It is this overlap, however, that enables the role to be cost-effective. The CNS/NP assumes responsibility for tasks normally done in the NICU by paediatric residents or clinical assistants. The sources of funding for the CNS/NP salaries reflect this form of substitution. Because CNS/NPs fill a gap in staffing, they are not perceived by physicians as a threat. On the contrary, the CNS/NPs are viewed as a precious resource. There have been minor conflicts with respect to competition for clinical experiences among the CNS/NP students and the paediatric residents, but these were resolved in an equitable manner.

As stately previously, the randomized trial involving CNS/NPs demonstrated that parents were satisfied with the care they and their infant received from that group.[23] The role of the CNS/NP is explained to parents in a number of ways. Explanations include written information, which is usually distributed to parents when their infant is admitted to the NICU, as well as on an individual basis by the CNS/NP and medical staff when parents first visit the unit. The author is unaware of any anecdotal instances where parents have requested that CNS/NPs not be involved in their infant's care. Parents seem to have accepted the role without reservation and, in most instances, are happy to communicate exclusively with the CNS/NP regarding the medical care of their infant. The neonatologists, therefore, have more time to devote to the parents of infants who are at high risk of death or significant disability.

The need for NNPs in Ontario continues as the level of acuity in NICUs increases, as more downsizing occurs in residency positions, and the use of foreign graduates in NICUs is restricted. Although the need for the CNS/NP was the impetus for the role implementation initially, it also constitutes a threat to the role at the present time. This threat comes in the form of the introduction of hospital-based programs which provide a 'quick fix' approach to staff shortages. Nurses who are not interested in pursuing further formal education seem quite prepared to assume responsibility for medical tasks with only informal training. Such training is not transferrable to another hospital or accepted for credit toward a university degree. It does, however, provide relief to medical staff who are increasingly burdened with the day -to-day care of critically ill neonates. This contribution to health care comes at a high cost to the profession and jeopardizes the advances made by other nursing colleagues. Without legislation to standardize eligibility requirements for the NNP role, the spread of hospital training may continue as long as nurses are willing to participate in the programs and hospitals are prepared to utilize them in NICUs. In order to prevent any undermining of the work that has been done in the province with respect to the NNP role, nurses must make their political voices heard through their professional organizations. They must respond in writing to any publication of such training programs and support those programs which adhere to the current recommendations by the professional organizations. The future of advanced practice nursing in Ontario and in Canada is in the hands of the profession, as long as we have the strength to carry it forward.

... In Paediatric Oncology...

Barbara Love

My transition from paediatric nurse intensivist to public health nurse to paediatric nurse practitioner was surely an exercise in happenstance. I had worked in a paediatric cardiac intensive care unit in Europe and returned to Toronto, laden with experience and enthusiasm. A brief stint as a public health nurse titillated my desire for independent or at least collaborative practice, and a chance perusal of the national newspaper directed me to a newly opened University Health Science Centre and a position in child-and-family care.

The physical site was quite 'avant garde' in the early 1970s-a basic adaptable shell amenable to change with sculpted walls, patient rooms overlooking windowed courtyards, an esplanade, and a mission to create a community-like atmosphere.

But more evolutionary was the philosophical conceptualization of care. Collaborative professional care meant that the child and family were pivotal team members. There was a healthy acknowledgment of individual professional competencies, and an attempt to recognize similar theoretical frameworks and to avoid duplication of skills.

As a paediatric ambulatory clinic manager and nurse practitioner, I worked with a variety of secondary paediatric clinics: orthopaedics, general surgery, genetics, haematology-oncology, and general paediatrics. Though the depth and breadth of my interaction varied with the individual team, their need, and my knowledge and skill base, some of the consistent role functions included health assessment (obtaining history, completing and documenting physical examination), collaborating with the health care team to define the problem and develop a plan of action, participating in that plan as required, evaluating outcomes at predetermined intervals, and submitting regular written and oral feedback to the referral source. Program variations ranged from collaborating on the development of a preoperative care package, to sitting with the families of dying children, to collecting blood samples of first-generation relatives of genetically compromised children in the community, to school reintegration visits with chronically ill children and their families. A large part of the knowledge base required for the expedition of this evolving role was acquired through front-line apprenticeship, attending workshops and formal certificate programs like the Clinical Behavioural Science Program offered through the Department of Psychiatry, reading voraciously, and actively exchanging information with other health professionals-and perhaps most importantly were the lessons taught daily by children and their families.

While clinically based at this site, I studied formally for my Master's in Health Science and thus obtained the credentials to function as a clinical nurse specialist (CNS). This was the only viable advanced practice allocation sanctioned by the provincial College of Nurses. The term Nurse Practitioner was still not recognized by the College, and the title Paediatric Nurse Practitioner (PNP) seemed aeons away. However, my peers, fellow health professionals, and management used the 'nomer' PNP to define the role being practised in the institution's ambulatory units.

In many ways, this position was extremely satisfying. With a diversely prepared, committed professional team, I could share comprehensive holistic care. The academic environment supported inquiry and excellence in practice, and continuity ensured involvement from diagnosis to discharge. But no system is fail-safe, and this site was subject to the whims of the institution, the fundings by the Ministry of Health, and the constituency and climate of the individual teams.

I subsequently spent several years at a tertiary care paediatric institution hired as a clinical nurse specialist. Faced with the increased complexity of health care needs in the late 1960s, this hospital's administration began to examine the role of the CNS, believing that the needs of patients and staff might better be accomplished by someone with this focus. It was determined that the CNS would assist the child and family in coping with hospitalization and illness through involvement in all aspects of care (i.e., physical, emotional). The anticipated by-product would be quality nursing care, and increased learning by all team members with whom the specialist worked. The CNS would function as a role model in assisting nurses to give individualized care to patients. She/he would provide in-depth patient care to a small, select patient population. This role model approach would encourage better learner integration and application of concepts.

Childbearing and a move to another provincial site precipitated another career change. My formal academic teaching positions in undergraduate and graduate nursing education with two different universities entailed both tutoring about, modelling of, and evaluating many of the roles to be adopted by student clinicians. Working with undergraduate students in paediatrics, I had the opportunity to see the novice practitioner struggle to obtain basic skills and integrate some rudimentary theory into practice. Registered nurses returning for a baccalaureate degree often bring an experiential base but seek the theoretical framework to extend their practice into a more evidence-based level. Nurses returning for a graduate degree, especially the experienced clinicians, are routed for an advanced practice allocation, and they are eager to integrate their experiential base with more in-depth theory.

In addition, for the last ten years, I have maintained a private practice: collaborating on workshops on staff management for hospitals around the province, seeing clients independently, and collaborating to establish an independent professional telephone enquiry and problem-solving line. The workshops entail specialists, prepared in education, management, and health care at the master's and doctoral level, collaborating intra group to further our own theoretical understanding of conceptual issues besetting health care, and then consulting to individual sites with personalized learning packages. As an independent practitioner, I see individuals, couples, and families in therapy. My interventions often occur as a clinician hired by university-based, government-funded research grants. The therapy is carefully audited, and I am regularly supervised by clinicians considered experts in the field. Additional workshops supplement my clinical base. Finally, the entrepreneurial development of a professional telephone enquiry and problem-solving line was enacted with six colleagues and provided consultative employment for forty clinicians prepared at the master's and doctoral level.

My experience in independent practice leads me to believe that the time is ripe with opportunities for creativity but also rife with problems of at least a legal and fiscal nature. The 'right-sizing' of health care institutions will encourage collaborative alliances that will help to redefine health care in this province.

At some point during my professional practice, I began to realize that individuals (clients, nurses, and other professionals) in many ways determined the role description of the advanced practice nurse.

Calkin's model of advanced nursing practice delineates levels of 'human responses' to which nurses, depending on their experience, are able to respond.[30] Calkin postulated that while the novice nurse attends to a normal distribution of responses (i.e., the centre of a bell-shaped curve), an experienced nurse is able to identify and intervene using a wider distribution of responses (i.e., those distributed on either end of the curve). Calkin suggested that experience and intuition provide the basis for the variance. The advanced practice nurse, by virtue of their clinical and academic preparation, is better prepared to identify and respond to the wider response distribution.

It is my belief that the expanded nurse role can be actualized by a motivated, prepared nurse with extended preparation at the undergraduate level and with continuing education credits. The actualized nurse practitioner programs have shown that primary care graduates can effectively and efficiently meet the needs of the population in urban and rural settings.[31]

My concerns are with specialty areas and requests that have traditionally fallen in the category of advanced practice education, research, and consultation. My own focus, paediatric haematology-oncology, is a case in point.

The term 'clinical nurse specialist' dates from 1938 when nursing educators at Teacher's College, Columbia University attempted to conceptualize an advanced level of nursing practice based on scientific theory.[32] Despite these early beginnings, preparatory programs were not initiated for another ten years, and this usually took the form of a minor in nursing specialty areas like administration or education. The dearth of available positions for experts in clinical practice necessitated this educational practicality. Historically, then, clinical nurse specialists were hired to accommodate the established hierarchy, and they had primary responsibility for staff development, unit management etc. Actual nursing practice was a vicarious sideline assumed by clinicians who were less knowledgeable and less experienced.

Nurse educators, recognizing a need to improve standards of nursing practice, began incorporating programs into the master's level curriculums of the 1950s and 1960s. By the late 1950s the clinical nurse specialist role was being implemented in various health settings.

The First National Cancer Nursing Society Conference was held in 1973 and led to the development of the Oncology Nursing Society, an organization that promoted the highest possible education standards for oncology nurses. The tenet incorporated into the Oncology Nursing Society Standards for Advance Practice in Oncology Nursing is that the specialist, through graduate level education, has become an expert in a defined area of knowledge and practice in a select clinical area of nursing.[33]

So, in many ways, the development of the specialist nurse practitioner role and the clinical nurse specialist have paralleled each other. Despite their early beginnings, confusion still exists around role interpretation and expectations both within and external to the profession. This is, in part, attributable to incomplete or absent educational preparation, lack of role models, and non-existent job descriptions. The undefined nature of the role has led to confusion, frustration, and resentment on the part of community and hospital nursing administrators, nursing staff, other professionals, and the public at large which has, in turn, hampered the rate and uniformity of the implementation of the roles.

At this point in time in Ontario, the child battling cancer could interact with a nurse who has:

1. a college diploma and no extra paediatric oncology preparation;
2. a baccalaureate degree and no extra paediatric oncology preparation;
3. a baccalaureate degree and an NP designation with no extra paediatric oncology preparation;
4. a college diploma with extra paediatric oncology preparation through apprenticeship and/or formal programs;
5. a baccalaureate degree with extra paediatric oncology preparation through apprenticeship and/or formal programs;
6. a baccalaureate degree and an NP designation with extra paediatric oncology preparation through apprenticeship and/or formal programs;
7. a master's degree in nursing or an affiliated field with no extra preparation in paediatric oncology but with advanced preparation in a relevant specialty (e.g. adolescent mental health);
8. a master's degree in nursing or an affiliated field with advanced preparation in paediatric oncology; and
9. a master's degree in nursing or an affiliated field with advanced preparation in paediatric oncology and an institution-sponsored attendance at a NP program.[94]

Designates 3, 4, 5, 6 might be functioning in expanded capacities. They could be approved by the College of Nurses and prepared by their institution to intercede in specific capacities. But only individuals 7, 8, and 9 will function in advanced paediatric haematology-oncology practice-as practitioners, educators, researchers, and consultants. And only nurses prepared at level 9 and sponsored by their institution can diagnose, order tests, and prescribe treatment under the supervision of a physician. Present licensing prohibits designate 9 from functioning independent of her/his own institution.

In many ways the future of the paediatric haematology/oncology advanced practice nurses will follow the emerging health care patterns. The present provincial plan seems to be to 'downsize/rightsize' large tertiary care institutions and move less ill children to peripheral hospitals in the child's home community. In the past, these sites may have managed clinical oncology issues like fever and neutropenia. In the very near future, they may be handling maintenance chemotherapy. Furthermore, one of the large metropolitan institutions is proposing to investigate the administration of chemotherapy in the child's home.

Multiple health care trends are impacting on the role of a paediatric oncology advanced practice nurse (POAPN). These include the global issues of inflation and increased cost of health care, an advanced nursing practice reimbursement system, the shift in practice site (inpatient to outpatient, in-house to community, tertiary to community hospital), the accelerated consumerism in health care, and an accentuated need for client education. In addition, there are cancer-specific issues: an increased use of technology in cancer care, including an increased knowledge of symptom management and earlier detection and cancer prevention efforts, the chronicity of cancer, its rehabilitation, and the incidence of late effects.

How do these issues specifically impact on the POAPN role? Let's examine some of the issues from the various role perspectives. Relevant to the practitioner part of the role, knowledge of technical advances and maintenance of current clinical skills is critical for front-line practice. Role delineation (credentials and role development) and development of practice standards are essential for internal and external accountability. Public and administrative purse strings will require economic justification for the role and appraised cost effectiveness. Additionally, collaborative or competitive practice among health practitioners may determine practice modalities.

Research issues relevant to the POAPN include time constraints, funding, role development including proficiency in critique and computer literacy, interventions related to new treatments, and administrative support for research.

Consultation issues might be patient-centred (responsibility for clinical management of a specific patient, such as nausea control with chemotherapy), program-centred (focusing on planning, development, and evaluation of oncology programs), or case-focused on difficult case management issues (outpatient management of hypercalcemia).[35]

Regarding independent practice, it behooves the practitioner to seek legal assistance before establishing practice. What may seem the best legal structure for practice may in fact be prohibited by the professional body (eg. incorporation), or may be the test case.

Over time, the focus of nursing research has shifted from who advanced nurses were, to what advanced practice nurses did, to what the outcomes were for the recipients of the nurses' care.[36] The former two issues have been defined in a rudimentary form in Ontario, but the latter still bears investigation, and future models of care seem curiously absent.

Additionally, research needs to be done to identify the patients who will benefit most from direct/indirect POAPN consultation. It is also critical to determine the appropriate ratio of novice to experienced to advanced practice nurses within a given limit and to approximate nurse-to-patient ratios while factoring in needed levels of expertise.[36]

It behooves those who diagnose problems to participate in the problem-solving process so specific strategies might be developed to overcome these aforementioned barriers within core curriculums. These might include focusing on knowledge and skills in organization, management, and administration which include change theory, use of power and leadership, role development, clinical skills and competencies, research skills, and awareness of health care policies.[37]

Administrative support structures needed to implement and support the role include role support and valuing by hospital administration, financial commitment for the role, role delineation (i.e., staff vs line in the organizational structure, including the authority to implement change), support for research and professional growth/continuing education, clarity/accuracy of job descriptions of POAPN, and peer review/peer support groups.[38,39]

Major factors influencing nursing and health care today are scientific, technological, and societal. Increasing sophistication of biomedical technology (i.e., diagnostic procedures, surgical intervention, transplantation, and chemotherapeutic interventions) is not for the faint of heart, and societal factors like consumerism, access, and cost may determine the direction of advanced practice.[40] I face the future hopefully and believe that creative and innovative times are ahead. I also firmly believe that nursing is becoming proactive in seeking solutions to the problems.

... In Mental Health...

Anna Giallonardo and Rita Schreiber

With the changing health care system, there is increasing interest in the role of the nurse practitioner in various settings as a way of expanding service delivery. This is particularly the case in mental health, where a number of factors make adoption of the role desirable. Nursing has long had an important role in the care of the mentally ill, and the development of advanced practice nursing roles is a natural progression, both from the perspective of service delivery and in terms of professional growth of individual practitioners.

Alphabet Soup: The MHN, MHCNS, and the MHNP

At present, there are three major types of professional registered nurses practising in various capacities in mental health. The Mental Health Nurse (MHN) is a nurse with a basic education at the baccalaureate, or in some cases, the diploma level. These registered nurses have gone to school from 2.5 to 4 years. They have the knowledge and skills to provide comprehensive nursing care to individuals experiencing a wide spectrum of health-related issues, including those with emotional and mental difficulties. They can assist people with problem solving, and developing coping strategies to deal with such issues as grief, loss, and anger. They have a basic understanding of communication skills, and can interview and engage in basic counselling and crisis intervention strategies. They are knowledgeable about group dynamics and teach people in groups and as individuals about how best to manage their health concerns.

The MHN, as a general registered nurse (RN), works collaboratively with other members of the health care team, and has a relatively circumscribed area of practice. Her/his knowledge and skills in areas such as advanced psychotherapy, and group and family therapies are limited. Although the MHN administers and monitors the effects of medication and teaches her/his clients about it, she/he does not prescribe medication. In these ways, the MHN, prepared at the basic level of entry into the profession of nursing is able to provide the full range of nursing care, but is not educationally prepared to perform more advanced skills. In the U.S., the MHN with a baccalaureate in nursing is eligible for certification at the generalist level in psychiatric-mental health nursing.

An Advanced Practice Nurse (APN) in psychiatric-mental health is a registered nurse with advanced education in psychiatric nursing and supervised clinical training at the master's level. APNs who have title protection practise their clinical specialty under the rules and regulations of the regulatory body in the geographic area in which they are registered or licensed and employed. In some jurisdictions, APNs have prescriptive authority, and they are able to receive direct or third party reimbursement for their services. The role of the APN is multifaceted and may include clinical practice, education, consultation, administration, and research. The client care provided by APNs focuses on health promotion and living with limitations rather than on any illness per se. APNs may be employed in a variety of settings that include hospitals, clinics, community health centres, physician offices, and independent practices.

There are two advanced practice nursing (APN) roles in mental health: the Mental Health Clinical Nurse Specialist (MHCNS) and the Mental Health Nurse Practitioner (MHNP). Both the MHCNS and the MHNP can perform everything the MHN can and more. Programs that prepare MHCNSs and MHNPs have similar curricula.[41] APNs in mental health study psychological and developmental theories, psychosocial rehabilitation, group and family therapy, and psychopharmacology. The MHNP may also have additional course work in advanced physical assessment, differential diagnosis, and neuropsychiatry. As well, they are trained to deal with specific clinical issues such as sexual abuse, women's mental health, and addictions. Williams and Valdivieso [41] conducted a survey that compared the activities of CNSs and NPs and concluded that "CNSs spend significantly less time on direct care and more time on education, consultation, research, and administration than did NPs." NPs in this study spent 63% of their time on direct care. The employment setting was cited as the major influence on the amount of time APNs in mental health spend on various activities.

Clinical Practice of the MHAPN

In this section, we will present a selection of role/setting/clientele combinations, illustrating how an MHAPN, whether a CNS or an NP, could meet client needs. We use the term MHAPN to indicate the generic advanced nurse practitioner in mental health.

It is important to understand that, at the time of writing, NPs are not legally recognized in Ontario. An estimated 250 NPs working in the province are working without title protection. Understanding the legal possibilities will provide a context for full implementation of the APN roles in mental health. The role of the nurse practitioner (NP) in mental health varies with the setting and with the patient population. Because the role has yet to be developed to its fullest potential, there is significant room for creativity and diversity.

The Role of the MHAPN in Acute Care

The role of the MHAPN has not yet been fully developed in acute care settings in North America, although there is a significant need for this role. MHAPNs in a hospital setting may work in a mental health program or in an emergency department where they conduct mental health assessments, and if necessary, admit patients to inpatient or outpatient services. In general hospital settings, there are relatively few people qualified (or comfortable) to conduct mental health assessments, so that the MHAPN is a valuable asset in determining who needs to be admitted for intervention, and who can best be helped in a less intensive environment.

The MHAPN designs and implements a comprehensive plan of care and initiates the appropriate psychotherapy, group, and/or family therapy. In addition, the MHAPN is skilled in conducting physical examinations and can order any diagnostic tests needed to assist in formulating a diagnosis. The MHAPN prescribes and monitors the treatment regimen, including management of any psychopharmacological interventions. As appropriate, the MHAPN works with the client and his/her family to determine the best plan for discharge. As members of an outreach team, MHAPNs can provide community-based home care. In these ways, they can provide not only comprehensive holistic health care in an acute care setting for individuals and families with mental and emotional difficulties, but ongoing intervention in the community as well.

The Role of MHAPN in Psychiatric Rehabilitation

Psychiatric rehabilitation (PR) is a systematic process of assisting persons with severe and long-term psychiatric disabilities to obtain the skills and supports they need to be successful and satisfied in their community of choice.[42] The distinction is often made between treatment, which focuses on management of the signs and symptoms of illness, and rehabilitation, which focuses on the skills and supports needed for living. Nurses are among a variety of care providers who work in psychiatric rehabilitation settings, yet they can be marginalized into the limited role of administering treatments and medications.[0] Nonetheless, many nurses working in rehabilitation settings see the need for an advanced practice nurse in their setting. The mental health advanced practice nurse (MHAPN) can bridge the gap and provide both treatment and rehabilitation for persons with severe and persistent disabilities, bringing a holistic perspective to their care.

As an advanced practice nurse, the MHAPN has the knowledge and skills necessary to assist the individual with severe mental and emotional problems to move towards wellness. The MHAPN understands the principles and practice of psychiatric rehabilitation, as well as having a thorough knowledge of the social, spiritual, environmental, and physiological issues relating to mental illness. The MHAPN is capable of establishing a long-term relationship, assisting clients to problem-solve and explore their understanding of health, as well as promoting recognition and self-management of symptoms. As a councillor, the MHAPN assists the client to understand the relationship between interpersonal issues and his/her own mental, emotional, and physical state. In this way, a partnership is formed between the client and the MHAPN, and the client can learn to make informed choices about what treatment strategies are appropriate and acceptable.

In psychiatric rehabilitation, there is a long-standing shortage of qualified psychiatrists, making it an ideal setting for acceptance of the role of the MHAPN. Psychiatric rehabilitation is seen by some as unglamourous and unrewarding.[43] In many psychiatric rehabilitation settings, the psychotherapeutic skills of psychiatrists are underutilized, and their focus is often limited to biomedical concerns. The MHAPN can provide similar services as a psychiatrist with the additional benefit of providing highly skilled nursing care, as well as role-modelling and mentoring other nurses. The last two benefits could not reasonably be considered within the scope of practice of a psychiatrist.

MHAPNs in psychiatric rehabilitation are usually employees of a mental health facility or clinic. As such, they may work in inpatient or outpatient programs, or their practice may include both. As part of their role within the agency, they are involved with family and community support, and education about mental health issues. Because mental health issues can be stigmatizing, MHAPNs assist family members to adjust to having a mentally ill family member. In addition, they play a valuable role in community-based education, in order to build a community that welcomes and cares for its psychiatrically disabled members.

The MHAPN in psychiatric rehabilitation understands that change is a slow process and sees the rewards in terms of the impact on clients' lives. It might be that a particular client has successfully lived on his/her own for a year, or that another has learned some strategies to deal with his/her auditory hallucinations. Because nursing has historically made its biggest impact on people experiencing chronic suffering and illness, psychiatric rehabilitation is an excellent setting in which a MHAPN can practise.[43]

Independent Practice

Advanced practice nurses have long practised psychotherapy independently. Traditionally, clinical nurse specialists (CNSs) who have a master's degree with advanced preparation have been involved in individual, group, and family therapies. Many excellent CNSs have chosen independent practice.

The MHNP has similar educational preparation as the CNS in mental health and does much the same therapeutic work except that the MHNP tends to focus more on the practice component of the role. In 1990, the majority of NP programs in the U.S. were at the master's level, and by 2000, they will all be master's programs.[44] Advanced practice nurses in mental health in the U.S. have always been prepared at the master's level. The MHAPN assists individuals to gain an understanding of their interpersonal relationships and to develop effective strategies for dealing with them. MHAPNs help people explore family of origin issues such as childhood abuse, and the impact of past events on their current relationships. They can specialize in particular clinical problems, such as child and adolescent issues, functional somatic syndromes, substance abuse, eating disorders, or sexual abuse survival. Depending on the setting and the identified needs, the MHAPN is capable of focusing on individual, group, and/or family therapy. Likewise, the MHAPN may choose to do all three.

In recent years, psychiatric-mental health nursing programs have begun to include advanced psychopharmacology for CNSs as well as for NPs. In addition, the MHAPN may pursue extra course work in this area. The MHAPN is able to prescribe medications if these are warranted for treatment. This has the advantage that the nurse in private practice does not have to refer clients to another practitioner for medication management, a common practice for other psychotherapists who do not have prescriptive privileges. In this way, the MHAPN improves the quality of care by providing timely, continuous, inclusive service.

Other Roles of the MHAPN

MHAPNs integrate elements of education, consultation, and research into their clinical practice. As the primary focus of the MHAPN role is health promotion and disease prevention, MHAPNs spend the majority of their time teaching and counselling patients on a variety of topics. Other activities of the MHAPN include conducting staff development programs, mentoring students, and providing consultation services. MHAPNs assist MHNs and other nurses in the care of complex patients. As part of the multidisciplinary team, MHAPNs participate in a complex consultation network that includes other advanced practice nurses, MHNs, and physicians. Traditionally, MHAPNs have not emphasized the research component of their role. Numerous studies were conducted in the 1970's and 1980's that evaluated the practice of NPs. As the number of APNs with master's level preparation increases in Canada, APNs will be more qualified to collaborate with other health care providers in the identification, initiation, and implementation of clinical research projects. Table 3 summarizes suggested standards for MHNs at the basic and advanced practice levels.[45]

Barriers to Practice

There are several barriers that have affected the development of the role of the MHAPN. At present, the health care system remains based on the biomedical model, emphasizing treatment of illness, with less consideration or reimbursement for promotion and disease prevention. There is an imperative to do no harm, but no emphasis on encouraging patient autonomy or wellness. In order to fully implement the MHAPN role, biomedical dominance must be challenged.

Table 3A

Suggested Standards for the Mental Health Nurse (MHN)*

Area	MHN diploma or baccalaureate
Theory	o nursing theories o interpersonal theories o developmental theories
Data Collection	o biopsychosocial o mental status o emotional state o coping strategies
Diagnosis	o nursing diagnosis
Interventions: *Counselling*	o problem-solving (assistance) o coping with anxiety, loss, grief, anger o reinforce healthy behaviors and interactions o techniques = communication, interviewing, problem-solving, crisis intervention, stress management, relaxation techniques, assertive-ness training, conflict resolution, behavior modification o group dynamics
Health Teaching	o basic health teaching to individuals and groups re: coping, interpersonal relationships, mental disorders and treatments, physical and developmental needs
Social Skills	o physical, social, and self-control needs
Psychobiological Interventions	o medication administration, monitoring, and teaching
Milieu	o facilitating therapeutic milieu
Case Management	o coordination of services with community and other agencies
Health Promotion & Management	o teaching and identifying services for populations at risk
Evaluation	o nursing process
Peer Review and Collaboration	o peers = RNs
Research	o consumer o participant

* adapted from the American Nurses Association Council on Psychiatric and Mental Health Nursing Statement on Psychiatric-Mental Health Clinical
Nursing Practice and Standards of Psychiatric-Mental Health Clinical NursingPractice.

** physical examination by the person providing psychotherapy is highly controversial and may not be recommended.

Table 3B

Suggested Nursing Standards for the Mental Health Advanced Practice Nurse (MHAPN)*

Area	MHAPN (includes all of RN standards and adds:)
Theory	o psychological theories, psychodynamic theory, object relations theory, other (feminist, etc.) o rehabilitation theories o family theories
Data Collection	o complete psychiatric evaluation and history o use of specific assessment tools as needed o physical examination**
Diagnosis	o rehabilitation diagnosis o DSM-IV or ICD-10 where appropriate
Interventions: *Counselling*	o psychotherapy o group therapy o family therapy
Health Teaching	o specific education on identified issues, eg., sexual identity, family dynamics, etc. to communities and systems.
Social Skills	
Psychobiological Interventions	o medication monitoring, treatment, and prescription privileges o limited dispensing (ie, office samples)
Milieu	o designing and implementing therapeutic milieu o system and organization
Case Management	o consultation to agencies and other groups
Health Promotion & Management	
Evaluation	o outcome and process measures
Peer Review and Collaboration	o peers = CNS, NP, PhD, Psychiatrist
Research	o investigator

* adapted from the American Nurses Association Council on Psychiatric and Mental Health Nursing Statement on Psychiatric-Mental Health Clinical Nursing Practice and Standards of Psychiatric-Mental Health Clinical Nursing Practice.

** physical examination by the person providing psychotherapy is highly controversial and may not be recommended.

Human Resource Planning

The first NP program was launched at the University of Colorado by Loretta Ford, a professor of community health nursing and Dr. Henry Silver, a professor of paediatrics in the School of Medicine. Although a physician was originally involved in the initiation of the NP role, as a group, physicians have not wholeheartedly supported it. Physicians in the province of Ontario are the only health care providers in the province who receive third party reimbursement on a fee-for-service basis from the Ontario Health Insurance Plan (OHIP). Physicians are concerned that the use of NPs in primary care will have a negative impact on physician's roles, as APNs are potential competitors as deliverers of many services previously provided by physicians.

Although the number of physicians per capita is quite high in Ontario, there is a shortage of psychiatrists, particularly those willing to work outside the large urban centres. This has created a gap in mental health services in rural communities and towns outside large cities. A significant percent of patients who seek services for mental health concerns consult general practitioners, who may or may not be equipped to deal with the complex psychosocio-emotional concerns of the mental health patient. Recent research [46,47] has shown that, although many individuals consult family physicians about mental health issues, they may not find the help they need. Thus, the existing system lacks appropriate mechanisms for assisting individuals with special needs in mental health. The MHAPN is qualified to meet these needs.

With the reform of mental health services, there is a risk the chronic psychiatrically disabled population will be underserviced, as care is shifted to less skilled, non-professional providers.[48] This is not to diminish the valuable role that consumer/survivor initiatives can play in a reformed system. Rather, the intent is to highlight the continuing need for expert professional services as well. At present, however, trained health care providers such as MHAPNs are being replaced by generic workers, further decreasing accessibility of professional services in a vain attempt to save money.

There is a public perception that allowing more health care providers to obtain direct government funding (not necessarily fee-for-service) will overburden the already stretched health care dollar. The difficulty is that no estimation of the appropriate mix of professionals and nonprofessionals to deliver mental health services for the people of the province has been determined. In spite of major efforts to identify the mental health needs of the people, there has been a striking lack of health human resources planning to determine how best to meet those needs.

Funding of Health Care

The cost of health care per capita has increased at the same time that funding has been decreasing. Over the past ten years, the federal government of Canada has drastically decreased transfer payments to the provinces. This has left provincial governments to scramble for dollars in their attempt to maintain the same standard of service provision. In such economic times, the lure of reforming the mental health system can be appealing, especially when considering the high costs of running a system of mental hospitals. Although there are no data to support it, there is a widespread belief among policy makers that high quality mental health services can be delivered for less expense in the community. In this way, the numbers of beds for psychiatric patients has decreased, and patients are being discharged without sufficient development of community services.

Given the fiscal restraints, real and perceived, of the current environment, critics will object to the implementation of MHAPNs on the basis of the cost to the system. MHAPNs can bridge many of the identified gaps, and this can save money in the longer run, as unnecessary hospital admissions may be avoided. However, NPs are not mini-physicians, and promoting the role as potentially cheaper than the physician role would not serve nursing well.

Education

To date, there has been no funding for MHNP programs available in Canada. Programs to prepare CNSs in mental health are limited in number, and competition for admission is extreme. This has placed a heavy professional and financial burden on nurses who wish to become MHAPNs by attending programs in the United States. Individuals must assume the high tuition costs to purse an education that is not fully geared towards Canadian health care concerns.

In order to prepare sufficient numbers of MHAPNs, it will be necessary to have the appropriate numbers of qualified educators to teach and mentor students. To do this, we will need increased funding for graduate programs in mental health, both at the master's and the doctoral level.

To ensure that MHAPNs maintain their competencies, ongoing education will be necessary. Although the College of Nurses of Ontario (CNO) does not support the need for continuing education credits, the new quality assurance program requires that nurses demonstrate evidence of continued relevant learning.

As advanced practice mental health nurses have not been able to obtain direct reimbursement for their services, their ability to practise independently has been severely impaired. The setting exerts an influence on the nurse's ability to implement the role. For example, a large number of MHNs continue to practise in institutional settings that focus on pathology and illness. Such settings allow few opportunities and supports for clinical advancement and development into advanced practice nursing roles.

Nursing

The nursing community has not always welcomed the NP role, viewing NPs as operating outside of nursing in the world of medicine. This misunderstanding has led some nurses to oppose the role in favour of the more 'pure' advanced nursing role of CNS. However, it appears that the two roles have much in common in mental health settings, and may become one role in the future. It is essential that the nursing community recognize the MHNP as an advanced nursing practitioner. Without professional support, the role could lack the professional guidance needed to maintain a nursing identity.

In addition to distrust about the NP role, there has been confusion among nurses about the various APN roles. This is particularly the case in psychiatry, where many MHNs have assumed a variety of semi-autonomous roles in the community. As well, some CNSs in mental health, who focus on direct care, perform similar functions to MHNPs. The two roles of CNS and NP have similar educational preparation, so the confusion is understandable. The ideal way of handling this confusion is to view both practices as advanced nursing practice, focusing on the similarities.

Unlike physician groups, nursing organizations have a history of serious fragmentation and infighting. In order for the MHAPN roles to be enacted, the nursing community must move beyond these territorial issues and support the development of these roles, both within nursing and with the public at large. Williams and Valdiesvo [41] believe there is a need for both the MHCNS and the MHNP role.

Public Acceptance

The public is not well informed about the services that MHNPs and MHCNSs can provide. This is not surprising, as the public has very little idea about nursing in general. It is likely that, with some publicity, the public would accept MHAPNs as an appropriate provider of mental health services. Several factors need to be considered by MHAPNs in their efforts to educate the public about their services. The public includes several groups, each with its own learning needs, so that a variety of strategies should be developed. For example, information presented to some consumers of mental health services who have difficulties communicating should be presented in a simplified manner. In order to educate politicians, nurses need to understand the political process and become involved in it. Nursing organizations must advocate for nursing involvement in mental health human resources planning. In this way, the message can be promoted so that MHAPNs can be accepted as professionally autonomous practitioners in the mental health system.

There is much room for the development of the role of the MHAPN in the health care system in Ontario. The MHAPN can provide direct patient care, consultation, and education, all of which will promote health and well-being. The barriers to full implementation, however, are formidable, and mental health services are often the orphan child within the Ministry of Health, receiving attention only when there is a problem. If all the people of Ontario are to have access to professional mental health services and consultation, the role of the MHAPN must be fully adopted throughout the province. MHAPNs are able to fill the gaps in order to transform what Slavinsky [49] described as "the existing caring nonsystem" into a "system of caring."

The authors would like to thank Margaret Rhoads Scharf, MS, FNP for her assistance in preparing this section.

What have we learned about role development?

Chris Patterson

Role development is complex. The professional, legal, and political issues, which arise at any time, can impact on how the role is developed. Generally, the setting will have some influence on the types and intensity of certain factors encountered; however, many, if not all, will be applicable to any setting or specialty. The following are some of the challenges in role development and are reflected in the personal accounts of practitioners in the chapter.

Integrating into the System

The first task, when developing a role, is to plan an approach for successful integration into the clinical setting and institution. In the clinical area, this will require analyzing the environment for enhancing and inhibiting factors to the role, including specific structural and organizational characteristics of the site.[50] Formal and informal power structures and their potential influence on the role are determined, as well as the goals of the setting, and their fit with the NP's role. The political and negotiating skills developed in the clinical area will be useful in the political arena as NPs push toward integration into the health care system.

Gaining Administrative Support

Administrative support is essential for the longevity of the role. Therefore, it is useful to meet regularly with administrators and other professionals to discuss expectations, identify problems, and formulate plans.[51]

Developing Negotiating Skills

NPs must be able to negotiate and communicate effectively in order to develop their roles according to personal and professional criteria. Maintaining open lines of communication is important for ongoing role clarification and discussing the discrepancies among role expectations of the various parties involved.[52,53,54]

Defining Role Responsibilities

Identifying role responsibilities that are congruent with advanced nursing practice while still meeting the needs of the agency may not be as easy as one may imagine. Strategies to maintain balance in the role include establishing realistic objectives with administrators, nursing leaders, and physicians involved directly or indirectly with role development; prioritizing what role functions are appropriate at a particular stage of development; negotiating the timing of the introduction of new subroles; and communicating role responsibilities to nurses, residents, and other members of the health care team.[53,54]

Developing Professional Support Systems

Establishing professional support systems will not only require developing links to colleagues in the community and professional organizations, but an appreciation for the services of other health professionals, and strategies for promoting collaborative relationships.

Gaining Consumer Support

Educating consumers about the role of NPs can occur through informal mechanisms in the clinical area or through professional endeavors.

Establishing Practice Boundaries

Because of the legal restrictions on expanded role functions, establishing approval for expanded functions through appropriate professional and administrative channels, obtaining malpractice insurance, and seeking legal and professional advice are important to legal protection.

Having the Appropriate Educational Preparation

Obtaining the necessary education to fulfil role expectations and developing the new skills required are essential for safe and effective care. NPs must reassess their learning needs and seek out appropriate continuing education programs and certification programs to maintain their skills.

As the role progresses, certain barriers will be minimized or eliminated and new ones will be created. However, certain obstacles are long-term and cannot be resolved at the clinical level. These obstacles will require the support of politicians, administrators, educators, physicians, and nursing leaders within professional organizations. Many of the NPs in this chapter identified legal restrictions as a major barrier to the implementation of the role. In Ontario, participants in a needs assessment for NPs in primary care agencies identified barriers to implementing or expanding the role. The barriers identified by over 50% of all agencies were the following: unavailability of qualified NPs, lack of legislation to perform certain clinical activities, reimbursement, and unavailability of continuing education.[55] Therefore, role development must be viewed not only from a clinical level, but from a more global perspective which emphasizes the importance of political involvement

Chapter Four

...Is There Room for Both NPs and MDs...

Dr. C. Edward Evans,
Linda Jones,
Dr. Daniel Way,
Dr. Bosco Paes

... In a Family Practice Unit...

Dr. C. Edward Evans

"The relationship between the doctor and the nurse is a special one, based on mutual respect and interdependence, steeped in history, and stereotyped in popular culture."[1] So opens a paper, which revisits a description, written in 1967, of how doctors and nurses relate.[2] The author characterized the relationship as a "game" in which, "nurses were to be bold, have initiative, and be responsible for making important recommendations, while at the same time they had to seem passive ... [they] were to make recommendations, but their recommendations had to appear to be initiated by the doctor." The cardinal rule of the game was that open disagreement between the players had to be avoided at all costs. For many physicians and nurses, even today, those are still the rules. Part of the problem with the acceptance of nurse practitioners by both physicians and nurses is that, not only have the rules of the game changed in general, but the emergence of nurse practitioners has added a new wrinkle that both of the original players have difficulty coping with.

What has changed in the past 27 years? The concept of physicians' omnipotence has given way to broader recognition of their fallibility.[1] Although nursing is still a "woman's occupation in a man's world,"[3] the number of males in nursing is increasing, though at a much slower rate than females entering medicine. The image of the nurse as a handmaiden, waiting to carry out the doctor's orders without question, is giving way to that of a university-educated professional with knowledge and experience to contribute. In fact, one of the players (the nurse) has unilaterally decided to stop playing the game and instead is consciously and actively attempting to change both nursing, and how nurses relate to other health professionals.[1] Just to add to the confusion, onto the scene appears the nurse practitioner seemingly straddling the line between nursing and medicine.

Background

To put my views into perspective, it may be helpful to give some personal background. I graduated in medicine from the University of London, England, in 1960 and, after two years of hospital training in the United Kingdom and Canada, practised for ten years in a small town in rural Alberta, 120 miles from Edmonton. Since 1972, I have been a member of the full-time faculty in the Department of Family Medicine at McMaster University.

When I started out in the medical profession in England, nurses wore caps, crisp white bibs and aprons, and black stockings. They even had uniforms to wear outside of the hospital, where they lived in the 'Nurses' Home' under strict curfew. The head nurse was (and still is) called 'Sister.' It takes no stretch of imagination to see the strong historical connection with the nursing sisters of religious orders and the implied discipline that it involved, thus supporting Stein's contention that "to inculcate subservience and inhibit deviancy, nursing schools were for the most part tightly run, disciplined institutions."[1]

In those days nurses made beds, administered tender loving care, took patients' temperatures, measured pulse rates, gave subcutaneous and intramuscular injections, administered enemas and provided bed pans, as well as carrying out many other menial and, at times, degrading tasks. They did not draw blood, take blood pressures, set up intravenous lines, perform physical assessments, or have the temerity to make a diagnosis. Yet, as a junior house physician, most of the staff nurses, especially the sisters knew far more than I did. To survive in a very difficult environment, I would have been lost without their 'suggestions' and support, though I never admitted it-I was playing according to the rules without ever knowing the game existed.

During the ensuing years, I had great difficulty watching nurses encroach on my turf as a doctor. Taking blood pressures, for example, involved using two 'doctor's tools,' a stethoscope, and a sphygmomanometer. I had learned the skill with difficulty, now here were nurses doing 'doctor work' and, although I was loathe to admit it, doing as well as or even better than I did. I think I dealt with it by ignoring or even belittling the nurses' skills, but seeing a nurse carrying a stethoscope, the symbol of the medical profession, continued to irk me.

Looking back now, I realize that it was my own insecurity as a physician that was a large part of the problem. As I became more secure in my own skills, experienced clinically, and accepting of the accomplishments of my nursing colleagues, I was able to accept not only nurses' enhancing their role more easily, but I also realized the benefits for myself and my patients. I suspect that one of the reasons many physicians and nurses have difficulty accepting NPs is that they are not fully professionally secure themselves.

Historical Perspective

My first exposure to NPs was almost 25 years ago during my visits to McMaster before joining the faculty. The unit in which I worked had more nurses than physicians. The intention was that the nurses would function as NPs, making first contact with patients, although they had not had formal education to do so. Coming mostly from backgrounds in public health, they already had some of the necessary basic skills, and together we developed an expanded nursing role-exciting and interesting times! At about the same time, McMaster University was developing the Primary Care Nurse Practitioner education program,[4] culminating in the publication of the Burlington randomized trial of the nurse practitioner.[5] The investigators reported that NPs could safely manage 67% of the problems reported in a family practice.[6]

Since that time, I have worked with a number of NPs and for the past 18 years have worked, as co-practitioners, with the same person. We share responsibilities for our teaching practice, provide service for our patients, supervise family medicine residents and nursing students, and have been involved in research and education together. I find it difficult to see myself practising family medicine again without NPs, although, if I were in a fee-for-service environment, because of the inability to charge the health care plan for services of NPs, it would be virtually impossible to do anything else.

Before going further, in case you have not already discerned it, let me state I am strongly in favour of nurse practitioners in family practice (others will have to discuss their place in other situations and specialty areas). I believe they enhance patient care and broaden the scope of practice. I do not regard nurse practitioners as mini-doctors or physician assistants, but on the other hand, I do not feel that they can operate totally within the nursing model. I am in favour of nurse practitioners being independent professionals but opposed to them setting up in independent practice. I feel nurse practitioners and physicians working as co-practitioners can provide a quality of care that neither can provide individually with greater professional satisfaction to both. In the following pages, I hope to support at least some of these statements.

Political Perspective

There have been various reasons put forward for promoting the education of nurse practitioners, and they vary with the politics of the time in which they are proposed. In the early seventies, there was a concern that there would not be enough family physicians to provide medical care and that there was "inefficient utilization of highly trained personnel, particularly primary physicians."[7] But, by the early eighties, nurse practitioners seemed to disappear from the landscape-in fact, the McMaster program closed because of loss of funding. Now in the nineties, we have seen a resurgence of interest with the implication NPs can provide care more economically than physicians. In the United States, the argument has been put forward that primary care nurse practitioners are the only way in which the primary care to specialty ratio can be corrected by the next century.[8] Other suggestions have been that physicians are not good at preventive and wellness care, and NPs can do it much more effectively, leaving physicians to look after the more seriously ill and medically complicated patients.

Opposition

There has always been opposition from physicians for the reasons already mentioned-professional turf and boundaries, the 'doctor-nurse game,' professional insecurity, and so on. It is interesting to note, however, that the same physicians who are vehemently opposed to NPs working in major centres (where backup and consultations are readily available), see no problem with them working in remote communities where there is no immediate physician available. Nurses have been doing that in the Canadian North for years-long before the term 'nurse practitioner' was coined.[5]

In the present fiscal climate in Canada, it is understandable that physicians get nervous when governments suddenly become interested in a 'new' class of practitioner. Family physicians, especially, feel vulnerable. Family physicians are under pressure to work harder for less income-the threat to replace them with lower paid professionals threatens not only their livelihood but belittles the service they provide. Family medicine espouses the care of the whole person, including emotional and physical health, preventive care, and family care. If these aspects of care are taken from family physicians, they see themselves being relegated to the role of unfeeling technologists.[9]

The official bodies of medicine in Ontario (the Ontario Medical Association, the College of Physicians and Surgeons of Ontario, and the Ontario College of Family Physicians) give lip service to the concept of nurse practitioners, but then go on to raise barriers to their acceptance. This inertia reflects both the traditional relationship of physicians and nurses, and the concerns and fears of physicians at large.

Organized nursing has not been totally supportive either. There are those who insist nurse practitioners should operate totally within the nursing model, should shun the medical model, and should have all their teaching by nurses with no input from physicians.[6] The longstanding dictum that nurses should never make a medical diagnosis is a major stumbling block to progress in defining the nurse practitioner's role. Organized nursing is struggling with the medical aspects of the NP's role, and the direction advanced nursing practice should take in the future.

Opposition has been apparent from other professional groups. My experience on an advisory group for the Ontario Ministry of Health has made me aware that pharmacists are very uncomfortable with nurse practitioners' prescribing, as are laboratory technologists with test ordering, and radiology technologists with use of X-rays by nurse practitioners. Could it be that these groups resent nurses' achieving an expanded role while they are still limited to carrying out the orders of physicians and now nurse practitioners?

With all this opposition, do nurse practitioners have any chance of surviving? I believe they do. Not because of the various political justifications, most of them are untenable. For example, nurse practitioners do not provide lower cost care, because they spend more time with patients[10] and work less hours than physicians.[11,12] But nursing has changed and so have patients. The old image of nursing is giving way to that of advanced practitioners with independent duties and responsibilities to their patients.[1] Patient expectations have changed in that they are no longer satisfied with a symptom 'ticket' and leaving the office with a prescription; they demand explanations, health teaching, and answers to questions. Nurse practitioners, from their nursing background, excel in these areas.

Independent Practice

Why is there so much medical opposition to independent practice? The obvious reason is the fear of another provider in the market place competing for the same patients and the same health care dollars. Other reasons, though less obvious, are more important. While nurse practitioners may be able to manage two thirds of single patient encounters without physician consultation,[5] that is not the same as managing two thirds of the patients over time, as any one patient will have problems that need physician input at least one third of the time.[6] How would the nurse practitioner in independent practice deal with those problems? Either by referring to a family physician or general practitioner at extra inconvenience to the patient and extra cost to the health care system, or by referring to a specialist at even greater cost to the system. Nurse practitioners working in collaboration with family physicians are able to refer these problems to their physician colleague directly, and/or consult with the colleague without referring the patient.[13] The professional isolation of practising independently is removed, and patients can benefit from the differing areas of expertise of the co-practitioners.

Primary versus Specialty Care

My background has been with primary care, generalist nurse practitioners, not specialty-based nurse practitioners or clinical nurse specialists. It is with this group that my interest and experience lie. I have a feeling, but no evidence to support it, that one of the reasons a recent Ontario Minister of Health pushed for primary care nurse practitioners was because she felt that it would be easier to train them rather than their specialty colleagues because they would not have to know so much. This is a common myth! As with any health care provider in a primary care situation, primary care nurse practitioners may be faced with a wide range of problems ranging from trivial self-limiting conditions to acute life-threatening events. Patients are understandably not very skilled at triage, as a visit to any emergency department will testify. While family practice nurse practitioners do have the advantage of having knowledge of many of their patients over time, greatly improving their ability to assess these situations, nevertheless, it is extremely difficult to outline the scope of practice of a generalist. Primary care providers need a breadth of knowledge rather than the depth of knowledge required by their colleagues in specialty areas. In addition, as conditions present to these providers at a much earlier stage than to specialists, they are more difficult to recognize. Spitzer and Kergin stated in 1973 that "the exercise of clinical judgement is the characteristic that best discriminates the nurse practitioner from the individual who serves as a technician or managerial assistant to the physician."[14] So it is more important for nurse practitioners to augment their skills in data gathering and problem solving than attempting to produce long lists of protocols or cookbooks to cover every eventuality. This is another argument in favour of collaborative practice.

The Nurse Practitioner Role

Let me state that I am not going to attempt to outline the role or scope of practice of nurse practitioners in this chapter. For one thing, space does not permit it, and for another, I am not qualified to do so. I will, however, try to give some idea of how we operate in our practice, as well as give a brief overview of what appears in the literature.

Because we run a full-time teaching practice as co-practitioners, a good proportion of patient care is given under our supervision by the four family medicine residents attached to the team. Nevertheless, we both give direct patient care to maintain our clinical skills and to pick up the load when residents are overbooked, on specialty rotations, or on vacation. We each have a small group of patients that we see almost exclusively, mostly for the continuity of care experience that adds to the satisfaction of family practice and can so easily be lost in a teaching practice with multiple providers. We also try to take our fair share of difficult patients, both for division of labour and to role model for our residents.

Patients are booked with either of us, usually on the basis of availability, although the receptionist will, at times, triage some patients depending on the presenting problem. While we both may see any presenting problem, a mother with breast-feeding problems will more likely be steered to the nurse practitioner and an acute chest pain to the physician. When faced with a problem that is more in the area of the other's expertise, it is a simple task to either discuss the problem, consult, or hand over the patient-a manoeuver that occurs in both directions. We have learned a great deal from each other, over the years, while at the same time developing our own areas of expertise. I tend to deal with complex medical problems and procedures; the nurse practitioner plays a major part in wellness care, prenatal care, well baby care, and immunization. We both do psychotherapy and counselling and often do housecalls on our chronic shut-ins and nursing home patients together.

One frustration is that after seeing hundreds of episodes of otitis media or urinary tract infection, the nurse practitioner still has to come to me to sign the prescription, and should one of our few fee-for-service patients present with a problem, I have to either see them myself or forfeit the fee.

We do not use protocols. For one thing, as already discussed, there is no way we could develop enough to cover all problems. For another, I feel protocols demean the person for whom they are written. A well-educated, intelligent professional with good problem-solving skills and common sense is much more effective than someone who can follow a protocol by rote. We do, however, both use clinical guidelines, such as the recent Ontario Anti-Infectives Guidelines,[14] the Canadian Hypertension Society Guidelines,[15] or the newly published Drugs of Choice Formulary,[16] and other evidence-based documents.

In the recent planning activity around the status of the nurse practitioner in Ontario, there has been a great deal of discussion about their scope of practice. One proposal with which I strongly disagreed was that nurse practitioners should be limited to dealing with minor, short-term problems and not care for or monitor chronic conditions. I suspect that monitoring and managing stable chronic conditions, such as diabetes and hypertension, represents one of the main contributions to patient care of nurse practitioners at present and will be the area in which they make a significant contribution in the future. Nurse practitioners do a better job of monitoring stable chronic conditions than physicians, and the nursing model is ideal for this type of care. In fact, Nolan stated that while the medical model is the most appropriate, and indeed the one of choice when cure is possible, the application of such an approach is counterproductive in chronic illness.[17] Zuger, in a letter to *The New England Journal of Medicine*, stated that: nurse practitioners' preparation is probably more suitable than a physician for bonding with and educating patients, following treatment plans, monitoring signs and symptoms, and making the physician aware of untoward events.[18] It is my firm opinion that excluding nurse practitioners from chronic care would be a major error and do a great disservice to patients.

The alternative approach is to limit nurse practitioners' scope of practice to minor conditions only. This approach has been tried in a general practice in England.[13] Incidentally, this very progressive practice is situated in my home town and has strong connections to the Burlington practice of nurse practitioner randomized trial fame.[5] Dr. Geoffrey Marsh of Stockton-on-Tees exchanged practices with Dr. Patrick Sweeney of Burlington 25 years ago, and their younger colleagues have repeated the exchange since. It is interesting to see how differently the role of the nurse has developed in the two practices. Sister Dawes, in the English practice, a state registered nurse and state-certified midwife with extensive community experience, was trained in diagnosing and treating minor illnesses by sitting in with the duty doctor in the practice during his office sessions. She then was available to see patients requesting an urgent same-day appointment. She handled 86% of problems with no doctor involvement, but "did not do any opportunistic health checks nor deal with the hidden agendas that she detected but encouraged patients to make more appropriate and leisurely appointments at the special clinics in the practice or with their doctor." While the title 'minor illness nurse' is politically astute, in that it is less threatening than nurse practitioner and will cause far less apprehension in the nursing and medical professions, I cannot help feeling that a great deal of experience and useful patient care would be wasted by adopting this very limited approach to the expanded nursing role.

The Future

The immediate future may be difficult, but I believe that the development of the nurse practitioner is a natural and inevitable evolution of nursing and medicine. The present fiscal climate, although it has been a stimulus for governments to re-examine nurse practitioners, will hinder progress. As long as provincial medical plans will not pay for medical services unless they are provided by a physician, collaborative fee-for-service practice will not be economically feasible in this country-a fact clearly identified in the Burlington study over 20 years ago-and physicians will continue to oppose the acceptance of nurse practitioners. It will require a restructuring of physicians reimbursement mechanisms before nurse practitioners can be incorporated into family practice to any significant extent. The family practice involved in the Burlington trial subsequently became a Health Service Organization, in which the practice was paid, not fee-for-service, but a fixed capitation based on age and sex to look after their patients, a method of payment under which we also have practised for many years. This method enabled them to practise with nurse practitioners as co-practitioners without losing the 12% of practice income they would have lost under fee-for-service. As a bonus, they were also able to look after 22% more families than under the traditional model.[5] It is interesting to note that new methods of compensating primary care physicians are now very hot topics at many levels. The blended funding proposal of the College of Family Physicians of Canada is a case in point.[19] Should alternative methods of payment become widespread, nurse practitioners will come into their own.

The trend of patients being discharged from hospital earlier and earlier, and the necessity of managing more complex problems in the community, is putting pressure on family physicians, general practitioners, and community resources. Nurse practitioners, along with various community agencies, will make a key contribution to the care of these patients.

Conclusion

The views I have expressed here are my own, and I take responsibility for them. I am sure many medical and nursing colleagues will disagree with me. I hope so, because it is only by thoughtful debate and discussion that reasonable answers to these questions can evolve. It is unfortunate that politics often precludes reasonable and rational debate. To my medical colleagues, I echo the words of Jean Bayley of the Royal College Nursing, "nurse practitioners are ideally placed not to substitute for doctors but to complement them and extend the services they offer."[20] Our goal should be an "expert nurse complementing but not substituting for expert doctors, and together providing a better service to patients."[3] To my nursing colleagues, beware of casting physicians in the role of 'unfeeling technologists'[9] or attempting "to raise the putative expertise of the nurse practitioner by demeaning that of the primary care physician."[21] The development of the primary care nurse practitioner role is the responsibility of both professions, and collaborative practice cannot help but improve both patient and provider satisfaction.

In closing, I quote the final paragraphs from the paper with which I opened this chapter:

> In this new, more equal relationship, physicians need not abandon concern for the whole patient, nor do nurses have to quit nursing. Physicians' ability to remain technically expert while maintaining a humane attitude toward patients may depend in large part on the arrangements they work out with other professionals, especially nurses. Nurses provide for their patients' needs as they have traditionally done while enjoying the benefits of working more collaboratively with physicians and other health care professionals.

Physicians and nurses can both benefit if their relationship becomes more mutually interdependent. Subservient and dominant roles are both psychologically restricting. When a subordinate becomes liberated, there is potential for the dominant one to become liberated too.[1]

... In a Community Health Centre...

Linda Jones and Dr. Daniel Way

South-East Ottawa Centre for a Healthy Community (SEOCHC) is a community health centre governed by a community board, and mandated to serve primarily at-risk populations living in an area of 70,000. At-risk populations for our Centre include families receiving social assistance, youth, isolated seniors, and refugee and immigrant families. These populations live mainly in subsidized housing, in large tracts of townhouses, and in high-rise apartments.

As is common to community health centres, strategies for community development, health promotion, and disease prevention are integrated into the delivery of comprehensive primary treatment services through the use of an interdisciplinary team.[22] Primary health care positions include family physicians, nurse practitioners, community nurses, nutritionist, health promoters, foot care nurse and part-time chiropodist, consultant psychiatrist, and administrative and reception staff. Other services include counselling, social work, community development, support in the home for families and seniors, fund-raising, volunteer co-ordination, and multicultural liaison. Team members work with the client and one another to identify needs and develop solutions. The client may be an individual, family, group, or community. Consultation and/or referrals to external health and community services are made as indicated.

The Role of the Primary Health Care Nurse Practitioner

Within the centre, the primary health care nurse practitioner (NP) is fully utilized in an advanced practice role. In contrast to other nurses who serve mainly in a triage and support function, the NP acts as a primary provider. As part of the primary provider team, the NP works in close collaboration with the family physicians in a shared practice.

The NP works both in the clinic and outreach. In the clinic, individuals of all ages and families are seen for wellness and illness concerns. Functions within the clinic include health examinations for adults, adolescents, children, and infants; lifestyle counselling for issues such as nutrition, sleep, exercise, stress management, and smoking cessation; addiction assessments and referral; risk factor identification; and disease prevention counselling regarding osteoporosis, coronary heart disease, and sexually transmitted diseases. The NP is also involved in birth control counselling, pregnancy diagnosis, antenatal care for the first 28 weeks, postpartum assessment; supportive counselling in cases such as poor self-esteem, anxiety, situational depression, loss, and immigrant settlement issues; and life cycle counselling for parenting, adolescent sexuality, and menopause to name a few.

The NP also functions in an advanced curative role. Clients are seen for uncomplicated, episodic diseases such as otitis media, vaginitis, headaches, abdominal pain, rashes, muscle strains, and sprains. The NP is also involved in the early identification and screening of common chronic diseases such as hypothyroidism, hypertension, and arthritis. Once the client with a new chronic illness is seen by the physician for definitive diagnosis and initial management, the NP then resumes care for ongoing monitoring. As part of assessment, the appropriate laboratory and diagnostic tests are ordered using the physician's requisitions. Medications are prescribed, either through protocols or direct physician consultation. In addition, complementary therapies are well utilized, such as fluids and rest for viral illnesses, heat and cold for muscle strain, and imagery and massage for stress. Referrals to medical specialists are written by the NP in consultation with the physician.

Health assessments are holistic, with a broad focus on determinants of health such as educational level, isolation, poverty, employment, housing, as well as past family and personal health data, capacities, and resources. The NP may become directly involved in advocacy with an individual or family by making calls and writing letters to agencies administering family benefits, or indirectly by referring to external or the centre's social services.

The NP works in outreach. At our centre, outreach includes three hours a week in the housing projects and three hours a week of home visits for families and seniors. As directed by the community tenant association and community members, the role within the housing projects varies greatly: from seeing children in child care for runny noses, giving impromptu presentations at ESL (English as a second language) classes, seeing sick children home from school, teaching individuals their medications, or completing a group of camp physicals. Clients who are not registered with SEOCHC are seen for illness assessment in a nursing triage capacity with referral to their own family physician for definitive diagnosis. As for clients of the centre, they are seen and treated in the clinic.

Seniors and other housebound clients are seen as part of shared care with the physicians to monitor primarily chronic illness. Home visits for families who have difficulty accessing care may include infant exams, immunizations, or breast-feeding support.

As part of the large interdisciplinary team, the NP is involved in staff meetings and committees, and acts as a resource to the governing community board. In our centre, the NP is not directly involved in group facilitation, but assists the health promoters by making presentations. Work with the community developer may include direct participation in political action meetings, such as anti-racism or housing issues, or encouraging clients to become involved in issues. The NP may work closely with social workers on situations of family violence, or with the consultant psychiatrist for more complex mental health issues.

There are many joys associated with this advanced nursing role in primary health care. One is the increased autonomy of serving as an entry point to health care. Another is the long-term relationships with clients. The NP is one of the few in nursing who has ongoing contact with clients and families throughout their life experiences. It is also rewarding to work within the philosophy of community practice, which supports an environment of working with clients to care for themselves. As well, the interdisciplinary approach promotes 'healthy disrespect' of hierarchy and a mutual respect for our similar, yet diverse sets of knowledge and skills.

The Family Physician/Nurse Practitioner DYAD

Entering our tenth year, the authors have been involved in a successful collaborative practice. In our fifth year, we began to explore the reasons for our successful practice, in spite of the perception of animosity between family physicians (FPs) and NPs[23] Observations of our working relationship led to the description of the family physician/nurse practitioner dyad (FP/NP dyad), which was first published in July 1994.[24]

Previous descriptions of the nurse practitioner/physician relationship have considered the NP as a 'guest,' with the physician maintaining hierarchical control of the practice and 'lending' clients to the NP, or as a 'gatekeeper' with clients 'filtered' through the NP to the physician. A third description depicts the NP and physician in a 'parallel' relationship in which interaction is formalized and limited, with no recognition of the professions' overlapping scope of capacity. The most popular model was the team model, but it has its drawbacks when the 'team' has a captain and decisions are based on conformity.[25]

The best support for our believed ability to function actively was found in Freedman's article in which he described the underlying principle of the nurse/physician relationship as a "mutuality of concern for each other as well as for the patient."[26] He described three guidelines which follow from this principle:

1. Both parties must recognize the reality of the other's situation and respect efforts to integrate that within responsible patient care.
2. Relationships across these two professions should be characterized by respect for each other's perspective.
3. Mutuality of concern will lead both parties to recognize the necessary moral autonomy of the other.[26]

The FP/NP dyad is an alternative model of practice which involves the collaborative partnership of physicians and nurse practitioners in the administration of primary health care to a client population. A hypothesis of the model is that comprehensive primary health care is best provided through the collaboration of medicine and nursing.

The definitions of primary health care, nurse practitioner, family physician, and client used in the model are:

- Primary health care is the care that a client receives at first contact with the health care system to prevent or to solve a health-related problem. It is continuous and comprehensive care, including curative, rehabilitative and supportive services, health promotion, and disease prevention.

- The nurse practitioner is a specialist in primary health with advanced nursing knowledge, emphasizing client centred, holistic care, health promotion, and disease prevention. Nurse practitioners, in collaboration with the client, diagnose and manage human responses to actual and potential health problems, as well as in collaboration with the client and the physician, diagnose and manage diseases commonly seen in primary health care. Nurse practitioners practise independently and collaboratively within an interdisciplinary team.[27]

- The family physician is the medical specialist of the dyad, possessing a distinct body of knowledge appropriate to the needs of diverse patients in a changing society. The unique nature of the doctor-patient relationship is central to the practice of the family physician. Family medicine is centered on the family, in its various contemporary configurations, as the basic social unit. The discipline is health oriented as well as disease oriented. There is a major focus on optimal utilization of community resources. It emphasizes the importance of disease prevention and health maintenance, as well as curative and rehabilitative medicine.

- The client is the focus of primary health care activities. The client is usually an individual or a family, but can also be a group or a community. The concept of client replaces and expands upon the traditional concept of the patient.

The working relationship between FP and NP should not be hierarchical. It is based on mutual respect and on knowledge of one another's roles, functions, and skills. Practice should be collaborative, offering a full range of health care services; client-centred, involving a holistic approach and development of trust; and cost-effective, by allowing the appropriate provider to give a particular level of care.

A diagrammatic representation of the model shows the interacting relationship of the FP and NP in relation to the client and the primary health care system. (Fig 1) The intersection of the two 'provider circles' represents the area of shared practice.

Figure 1
Model of Collaborative Partnerships

FAMILY PHYSICIAN
Medical Specialist in

NURSE PRACTITIONER
Nurse Specialist in

PRIMARY HEALTH CARE

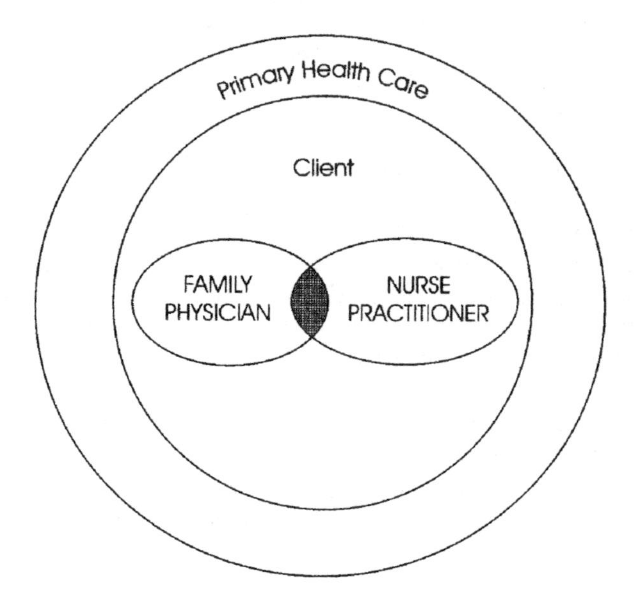

CLIENT can be an individual, family, group or community.

AREA OF OVERLAP equals the area of shared care.

SIZE of this area of shared practice is dependent on multiple factors:

1. knowledge and skills of the providers
2. client characteristics, needs, and wishes
3. work setting and its policies

Care is oriented primarily toward people and not disease, and places client involvement, health promotion, and disease prevention as priorities equal to disease treatment. Client care is not fragmented or duplicated. The client receives the benefit of the distinctive knowledge and skills of medicine and nursing, with a shared plan of care based on mutually agreed upon interventions and goals.

Since the knowledge and skills of both providers are utilized, care is efficient and more cost effective, focused on insuring the appropriate provider for the appropriate level of care. Clients are knowledgeable about both providers' roles and are known to both providers. Clients may remain with one provider or move readily back and forth between the nurse practitioners and the family physician to accommodate the client's preferences and health care needs. For example, some seniors wish to be seen by the FP only, whereas others with more complicated illnesses do not want to be referred but seen by the NP in consultation with the FP.

Some case examples help to illustrate this point. Previously, Helen had been seen by the FP in his solo practice. At first, Helen saw the NP for well women care and birth control counselling and monitoring. The NP consulted with the FP regarding the presence of an enlarged thyroid, and the appropriate diagnostic testing was arranged. The NP continued to monitor the function and size of her thyroid gland. When Helen became pregnant, she entered shared care. The NP provided antenatal care for the first 28 weeks, and the FP provided care for the third trimester and delivery. Helen and the infant remained with the FP for the postpartum and newborn periods, and then returned to the NP for well infant and women's care.

Betty, 86 years old and infirm, came from an inadequate care situation to live with her widowed niece and her family in a townhouse in a low-income project. The family was well known to the NP, who administered care to the niece, her children and grandchildren. The NP's initial assessment of Betty resulted in immediate referral to the FP because of an undiagnosed dementia and a large, undifferentiated abdominal wall. Examination revealed probable multi-infarct dementia, hypothyroidism, and metastatic large bowel carcinoma. Because the family wished to care for Betty at home, the FP and NP shared in palliative care for Betty and support of the family. After 18 months, Betty died at home in the presence of her family physician.

Model Utilization Under Current Legislation: Medical Guidelines

Under the previous *Health Disciplines Act* and now the *Regulated Health Professions Act* of December 1993, the advanced curative role of the NP was dependent on medical delegation.[28,29] Early in our partnership, we decided to develop practice guidelines (protocols or medical directives) for these 'medically delegated functions' - the diagnosis and management of short-term, episodic, or uncomplicated diseases and the early detection and monitoring of stable chronic diseases common to primary health care. If a client's problems fall within the guidelines, the NP will diagnose and prescribe without the need for direct physician consultation. The FP and NP will consult during the client's visit or at the end of the clinic day for cases in which a guideline requires consultation and/or referral, an unusual presentation of a common illness or response to treatment, problems not common to primary health care, the initial diagnosis and management of chronic diseases, or multiple, interacting health problems.

Our decision was to develop medical guidelines confined to that area of our shared curative practice rather than NP protocols or guidelines which would include the independent functions of nursing. The guidelines serve as a reference and not a 'cookbook' for medical practice. The NP must have and demonstrate the necessary knowledge and decision-making skills for the medical function included in the guideline. The guidelines present minimal expectations that should be met at all times, an important consideration for liability.[30] They clearly indicate to the FP what is expected of the NP, which removes the necessity for each new physician entering a practice to retest NPs. Accountable for their own practice, new NPs would review the guidelines and identify those they have knowledge and skills to perform. If there are deficiencies, a formal or in-service education program can be developed. The guidelines also communicate the overlapping function with medicine to funding agencies, administrators, and other members of the health care team. They help to differentiate the roles of the NP and other primary health care nurses. Finally, guidelines serve as 'standing orders' that allow the NP to care for most clients without the need for direct physician

consultation. Currently, the NP sees approximat
clients without the need for direct consultation o

The initial writing of the guidelines was a joint N
Existing references were adapted to reflect our practice.[31,32] Although time consuming, joint development was well justified, strengthening our understanding of shared curative knowledge and mutual respect.

Deciding which medical functions required a guideline was facilitated by an algorithm.(Fig 2) Areas of shared care in which guidelines have or are being developed include health maintenance; emergency care such as anaphylaxis and wound care; common primary health care disorders of the skin, eyes, ears, nose and throat, lower respiratory tract, cardiovascular, gastrointestinal, genitourinary (including sexually transmitted diseases), musculo-skeletal, endocrine, and haematopoietic systems; women's health (including family planning and antenatal care); and miscellaneous infections such as exanthem. The outline for each guideline includes a definition of the problem necessitating care, etiology, clinical features (signs and symptoms), laboratory and diagnostic studies, differential diagnosis, treatment, complications, consultation or referral, and follow-up.

Implementation of the guidelines involves authorization. A form is signed indicating approval of the agency, medical, and nursing staff for delegating the medical function. This form also includes a list of the NPs authorized to carry out the guidelines and a schedule for reviewing and updating the guidelines. Periodic joint review by the users is an essential part of the process for keeping the guidelines current and sensitive to the setting. Misuse of the guidelines would occur if external guidelines were imposed by administration or by one member of the dyad without joint review and adaptation. They would also be misused if they supported separate, 'parallel' practices without fostering mutual consultation and partnership.

re 2

To Determine Whether a Function Requires a Guideline

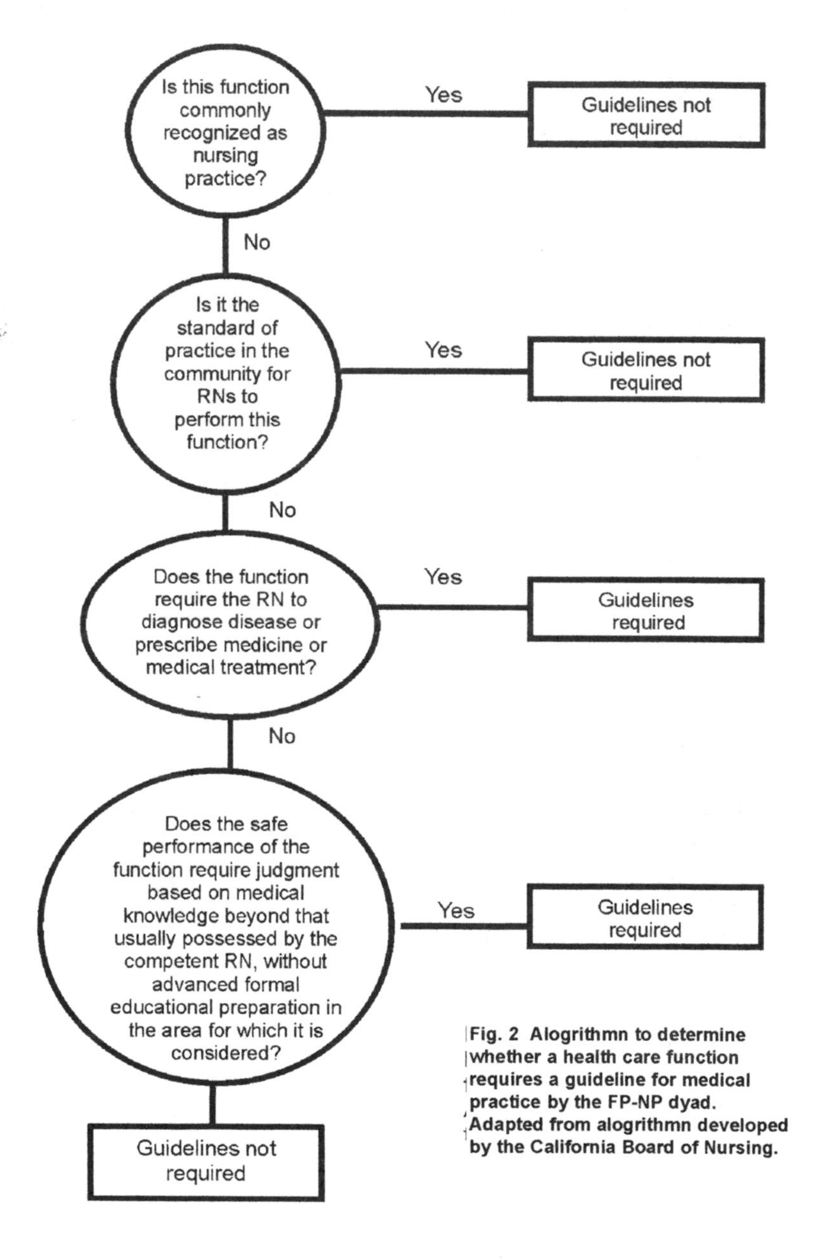

Fig. 2 Alogrithmn to determine whether a health care function requires a guideline for medical practice by the FP-NP dyad. Adapted from alogrithmn developed by the California Board of Nursing.

Our practice guidelines could be adapted for use by other FP-NP partnerships in other settings. The definition, etiology, clinical features, differential diagnosis, and complication portions could be standardized. The laboratory and diagnostic studies, treatment, and follow-up portions of the guideline might vary, depending on the setting. For example, because we work primarily with seniors and low-income families, the medications prescribed are limited to those in the Ontario Drug Benefit Formulary.[33]

Utilization of consultation and/or referral might also vary. NPs with formal educational preparation and/or years of experience may choose to consult with the FP rather than refer. It is essential to stress that the medical guidelines support the FP/NP dyad by clarifying shared curative functions and formalizing direct and indirect consultation. Freed from the need for constant direct consultation, time is used for mutual consultation to support holistic client care.

Effects of the NP Project on the NP role and on the Collaborative Model

NPs currently employed in community health centres (CHCs) have been either educated in the 1970s and early 1980s programs in Canada or American NP programs, or have received their training through experience without formal preparation. This current lack of standardization results in varied, and often limited utilization of NPs knowledge and skills. It is confusing for CHC boards and employers to determine liability and accountability issues. Therefore, they may choose not to utilize the NP's curative role. Without education standards, it is also difficult to communicate the role to consumers and to other health providers.

At the time, proposed legislative and regulation changes refer primarily to the *Regulated Health Professionals Act.*[29] In December, 1993, the *Health Disciplines Act* was replaced by the *Regulated Health Professions Act* (RHPA) with its listing of thirteen controlled acts. Of special importance to the NP were the controlled acts referring to communicating a diagnosis, ordering a form of energy (i.e. diagnostic ultrasound), and prescribing medications. These acts were primarily reserved for medicine and are not part of the scope of practice of nursing.

The extended curative function is essential to the NP role. In spite of growing emphasis on health promotion and disease prevention, the vast majority of Canadians seek primary health care when they are ill. The curative role allows the NP to serve as a point of entry to the health care delivery system. Once seen for illness, the NP is able to engage the client in health promotion and disease prevention strategies.

The extended curative role is dependent on the ability to formulate and to communicate a diagnosis, to order and to interpret the results of diagnostic and laboratory tests, to treat illness, to prescribe medications, and to refer to medical specialists. As part of the NP project, regulations would be changed to allow the NP, as a member of a new extended registered nurse category, to initiate the three controlled acts without the approval or supervision of the physician.[35] Without these extended acts, the NP would continue to require medical delegation--the physician must agree that the NP has the necessary knowledge and skills to initiate the controlled acts and agree to delegate these acts.

Educational standardization and legislative changes will clarify liability and accountability issues, allowing community health centre boards and employers to fully utilize the curative role of the NP as part of a comprehensive primary health care service. As an example, the role of the NP in outreach programs could be greatly enhanced. The NP would be able to more fully serve clients and would be free to collaborate with physicians outside of the centre.

Legislative changes that legitimize the NP role will benefit the collaborative role with the family physician. Many CHC physicians have been hesitant to work with NPs, as long as they were accountable for delegation. Collaborative partnerships between FPs and NPs would be truly based on equity, without one being accountable to or for the other. This equity will strengthen our current model, the FP/NP dyad.

Medical guidelines or protocols will no longer be necessary for medical delegation. Guideline development could focus on best practice guidelines for all primary health care providers, with emphasis on accountable and cost-effective practices.

The new education program began in September 1995 in Ontario. The request for regulation changes to the RHPA was reviewed by the Health Professions Regulatory Advisory Council, a public council mandated to advise the Minister of Health on matters of regulatory changes pertaining to all regulated health professionals.[36,37] Their final report, supporting legislative changes, was received by the Progressive Conservative Minister of Health in June, 1996. Eventually, the Expanded Nursing Services for Patients Act was proclaimed in Ontario allowing nurses holding an extended certificate of registration to perform certain acts.

Medical Response to the NP Project and to Proposed Changes in Regulation

Overall, there has been longstanding animosity towards NPs from physicians and their political organizations. The concept that many of the tasks performed by physicians may be done by another, less costly health professional, such as NPs, is inherently threatening to physicians from the perspective of job security and the belief that only medicine can make medical diagnosis, regardless of the condition.[38,39]

In Ontario, in 1995, this debate continued in the context of new regulations proposed by the Ministry of Health to give access to the three extra controlled acts under the RHPA to an extended class of registered nurses. The medical professions' animosity is apparent in the major arguments proposed by the three medical organizations in their submissions to the Health Professionals Regulatory Advisory Council (HPRAC). The Ontario Medical Association (OMA), the Ontario College of Family Physicians (OCFP), and the College of Physicians and Surgeons of Ontario (CPSO) presented their opinions on the utilization and education of NPs to HPRAC during the June 10 and 22nd public hearings. These reports offer an insight into the arguments that the medical profession presented in its opposition to regulatory changes in the scope of practice for NPs.[40,41,42]

The arguments of the OMA and the OCFP are similar. The OMA is the organized voice of Ontario's 23,000 physicians, recognized as their official 'negotiating' agent by the government. The OCFP represents FPs in Ontario and has its own political agenda, but has a more educational focus than that of the OMA. In particular, two arguments reflect their animosity.

The first argument is that independent NPs will be more expensive to the health care system in duplicating services, investigations, and prescriptions. They argue that NPs will be inadequately prepared to make appropriate referrals to other health care professionals, and this will result in higher, not lower, costs to the system.[40,41]

Physicians have traditionally interpreted 'independent' to mean practising in an autonomous fashion, (solo or in groups) without collaboration. In fact the use of the term 'independent' in the regulations refers to legal sole accountability to the College of Nurses for a NP's own action in diagnosis and prescribing rather than autonomy as medically defined. The term 'independence' used in the regulations means that medical delegation for the extended acts is no longer required. Nursing autonomy does not negate collaboration.

The intent of the Ministry of Health NP Project is to employ NPs in existing organizations and agencies. There is provision in underserved areas where no appropriate organization or agency exists for District Health Councils to be supported to establish independent NP practices.[34] Independent practice, in this context, would facilitate access to needed health care and not duplicate care. The Canadian health care system is not based on competition. Obviously, in times of fiscal restraint and rationalization of health resources, NPs will not be funded to establish independent practices in well-resourced areas. NPs working in collaborative practices, such as in CHCs, or with physicians reimbursed through alternative payment mechanisms outside the CHCs, will not add more expense to the system. Rather they will allow the more expensive physician resource to focus upon more complicated illness care.

The second argument is that evidence often cited to support utilization of NPs in Ontario is flawed. The Ministry of Health commissioned a report entitled, Utilization of Nurse Practitioners in Ontario, that concluded that NPs provide a cost-effective care that can be substituted for certain areas of medical service. This conclusion is based on American and Canadian studies.[43] Organized medicine refutes the claim, citing that:

1. The majority of the studies are American and their conclusions cannot be extrapolated to the Canadian situation. The American system is too dissimilar to make any comparison of NP utilization valid.
2. The Canadian studies used are 20 years old, and their results are not applicable to the current health care situation.
3. The claim for NPs' cost effectiveness is unsupported in the literature.
4. A major bias that was not accounted for in the studies examined was age and sex. The NPs in the studies were younger women, while the physicians were older men. They contend that the differences in patient preference and satisfaction could be accounted for by this bias.[40,41]

The CPSO, which is the regulatory body of physicians in Ontario, in its submission to HPRAC, chose to focus its comments upon questions about educational preparation to a much larger degree than the OMA or OCFP. In addition, there was concern about process problems related to the NP Project with lack of consultation by the Minister of Health with organized medicine from the start of the project. If such consultation had occurred, potential problems could have been avoided. For the College, issues such as the lack of a clear scope of practice from a medical perspective and of role clarification so as to prevent further fragmentation of the primary care system were problematic.[42]

Interestingly, all three groups declared support for the concept of an expanded role for nurses within primary care. However, the OMA and OCFP limited their support to what really amounts to enhanced physician assistants on multidisciplinary teams, where physicians fill the key leadership role. The CPSO position was more supportive of a collaborative model, where FPs and empowered NPs combine skills to provide better patient care.

The previous Ministry of Health of the New Democratic Party (NDP) government needs to accept responsibility for much of the animosity physicians have towards the NP project. They were in a position to encourage broad consultation on appropriate models of integration of these two primary health care specialists. They chose not to pursue such a course focusing on consultation with primarily nursing organizations in the defining stage and with groups of key informants, including medicine, late in the process.[44] The Ministry's lack of initiative in providing a primary health care framework had also hurt co-operation. Such a framework is essential if the goal to achieve an integrated, comprehensive, and efficient health care delivery system is to be attained. With a multitude of initiatives in health care service reform underway in Ontario, of which the NP project is only one, a framework would have been a major asset in promoting the consultation and collaboration which was lacking in this project.

Summary and Conclusion

We have focused on the role of the primary health care nurse practitioner within a community health centre setting, with emphasis on a model of collaborative practice, the FP/NP dyad. Under past legislation, the dyad was supported by the use of medical guidelines or protocols related to the medically delegated role of the NP. Under the current legislative changes in Ontario, medical delegation is no longer necessary for NPs to carry out their extended curative role, essential to their comprehensive practice. Collaboration is facilitated, based on mutual respect for each professions' knowledge and skills with no one provider being accountable to or for the other.

Family physicians and nurses are trained in a model of care which encompasses comprehensiveness and continuity of care. These attributes are complementary to collaborative practice. Once FPs can move beyond the animosity over the role of NPs in primary health care, they will realize that the last 25 years of family medicine training in Canada has produced physicians who are ideally suited to the type of collaborative model described in the FP/NP dyad. In Ontario, with the increased emphasis on encouraging health promotion and disease prevention, the family medicine and nursing models can mesh to fulfill these demands. The NP's strengths in diagnosing human responses, and in client education, counselling, and health promotion can be linked with the FP's strengths in medical diagnosis, treatment, and disease prevention, to offer effective and efficient client care.

...In a Neonatal Intensive Care Unit...

Dr. Bosco Paes

With the development of advanced educational programs, crises in physician staffing of intensive care units and severe financial constraints in the health care system, the scope of practice of nurse practitioners has changed considerably. NPs are now increasingly in demand in adult, neonatal and paediatric intensive care settings, and emergency departments. More importantly, with the implementation of cost containment strategies in the health care system in Ontario and the focus on community-based primary disease prevention and health promotion programs, NPs are striving for recognition and integration into primary care settings.

Role Development and Implementation

With the evolution of the NP role, registered nurses sought to advance their knowledge base and expertise, recognizing the need for upward professional mobility.[45] The move into the intensive care arena resulted in a change of educational programs from a hospital-based certificate level to university based master's degree programs and even training at a doctorate level, which has recently been endorsed by the Board of Directors of the National Association of Neonatal Nurses.[46] This has resulted in titling confusion, and controversy still exists as to whether the title of NP should be maintained for the primary care setting while clinical nurse specialist and that of critical care nurse practitioner should be reserved for those functioning in high-risk units. Figure 3 shows the overlap of roles between the clinical nurse specialist and nurse practitioner.[47] In neonatal intensive care, the National Association of Neonatal Nurses has agreed that clinical nurse specialist/neonatal nurse practitioner (CNS/NP) be appropriately used to delineate practice in the field.[48] For the purposes of this chapter, an NP is defined as "one who is able to use sophisticated knowledge, to demonstrate a high level of accountability to persons served and to teammates, and to assume roles commensurate with professional nursing preparation."[49] Nurse practitioners currently function in primary, secondary, and tertiary care settings, with the greater role emphasis placed on community-directed health services.

I have been involved in the development of the Neonatal Nurse Practitioner Program (NNP), the first of its kind in Canada, at McMaster University Medical Centre. Historically, the development of the NNP program stemmed from a request by the Minister of Health in 1980 that the Ontario Council of Administrators of Teaching Hospitals (OCATH) collaborate with the Council of Ontario Faculties of Medicine (COFM) to examine alternative staffing needs in teaching hospitals. This was in response to concerns expressed by OCATH and COFM over the effect which projected reductions in the number of Ministry of Health funded resident positions might have on the standard of patient care in teaching hospitals. A number of subcommittees were struck to examine alternatives to residents for provision of critical care services to patients. The neonatal subcommittee unanimously agreed that nurses, with appropriate preparation, would be capable of assuming responsibilities equivalent to those performed by paediatric residents in a supervised training program. In its summary, the neonatal subcommittee stated that the introduction of such a role would improve the standard of patient care, the quality of the teaching environment, and possibly the attractiveness of a career in neonatology for graduates of Canadian medical schools. The College of Nurses supported the use of the registered nurse in an expanded nursing role. Their report summarized studies which indicated that the level of care, interdisciplinary communication, and patient satisfaction all remained high where registered nurses had functioned in expanded roles. The OCATH and COFM committees recommended the development of pilot projects in specific areas of practice, such as neonatology, adult intensive care, and cardiovascular-thoracic surgery.

Figure 3
Clinical Nurse Specialist - Nurse Practitioner Overlap

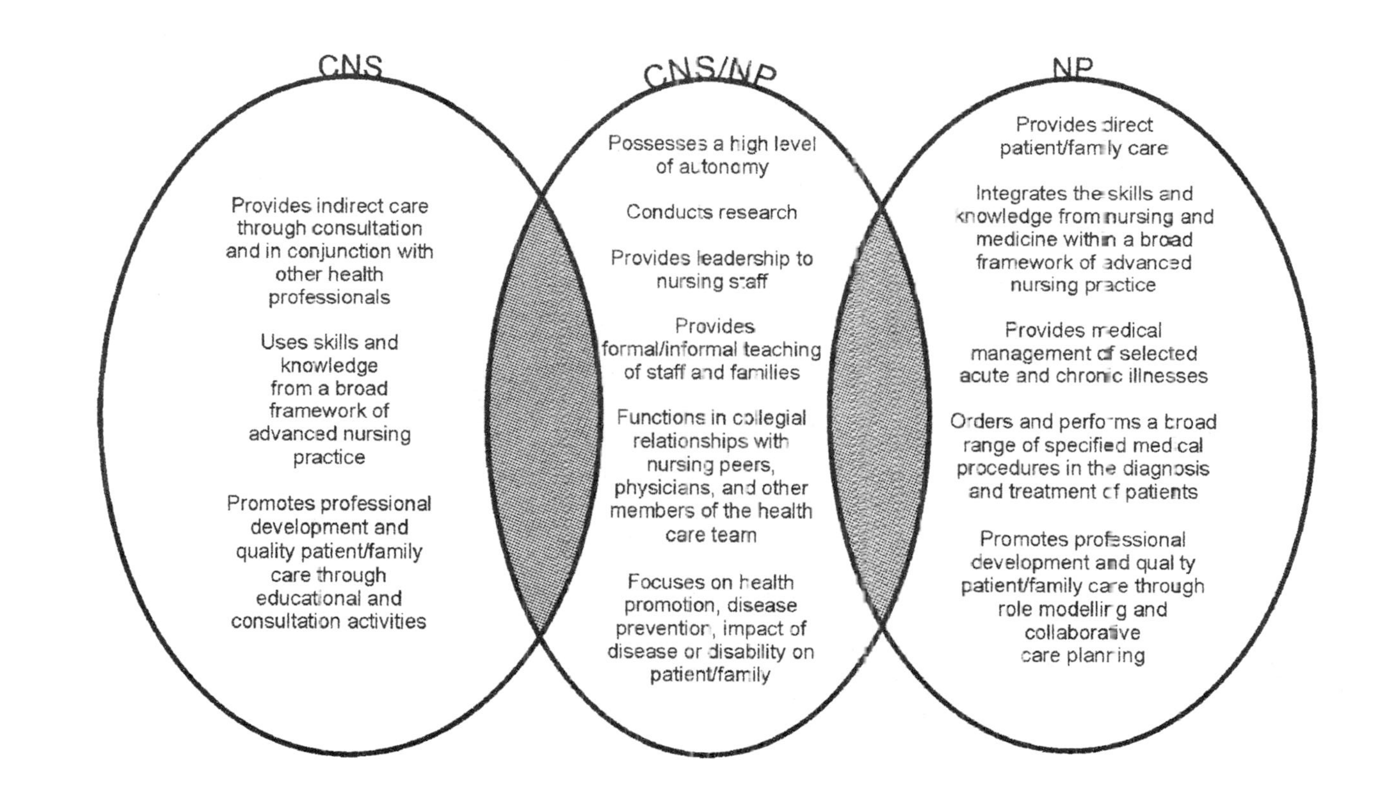

A research team at McMaster determined that there was a shortage of medical personnel in Ontario neonatal intensive care units and identified alternatives to alleviate this shortage.[50] The level of nursing practice with respect to clinical decision-making and general background knowledge in biopsychosocial sciences set nurses apart as the health care professionals who could best meet current needs, by providing the most consistent and best quality care. Further funding was utilized to define the NP role, determine the additional preparation required for the role, and obtain approval from nursing and medical professional organizations. The program evolved from a disequilibrium in the medical staffing of neonatal intensive care units (NICU) with the demand on health care services far exceeding the availability of medical personnel.

The role was developed encompassing a high level of professional performance, including technical expertise, independent decision-making, and leadership skills.[51] Neonatal practitioners assume responsibility for the care of an assigned number of neonates and, in addition, have educational, research, and administrative responsibilities. Approximately 70% of their time is devoted to clinical practice, which encompasses assessment, diagnosis, planning, management, therapeutic interventions, and ongoing evaluation of clinical care.[51] Educational responsibilities are directed towards the professional development of nurses in the NICU, undergraduate students in nursing and medicine inclusive of medical interns and junior residents. NPs act as a resource to parents and are actively involved in outreach educational activities in Ontario. They are specifically trained in research methodology, facilitating and implementing clinical trials which cross boundaries between nursing and medicine.[52,53] Lastly, neonatal NPs are actively involved in administrative activities directly linked to the NICU, the hospital and the community. The clinical practice is viewed as collaborative between practising physicians, neonatologists, and NICU staff nurses, with a significant overlap of skills and knowledge.(Fig 4) The philosophy of partnership de-emphasizes what is nursing and what is medicine in order to avoid territorialism and helps to consolidate the approach to clinical care. The NP is not viewed as a physician replacement, the role is a model of excellence which serves to "blend the medical and nurses aspects of care into a distinctive whole."[54]

Figure 4
Overlap of Skills and Knowledge in the NICU: Physicians and CNS/NPs

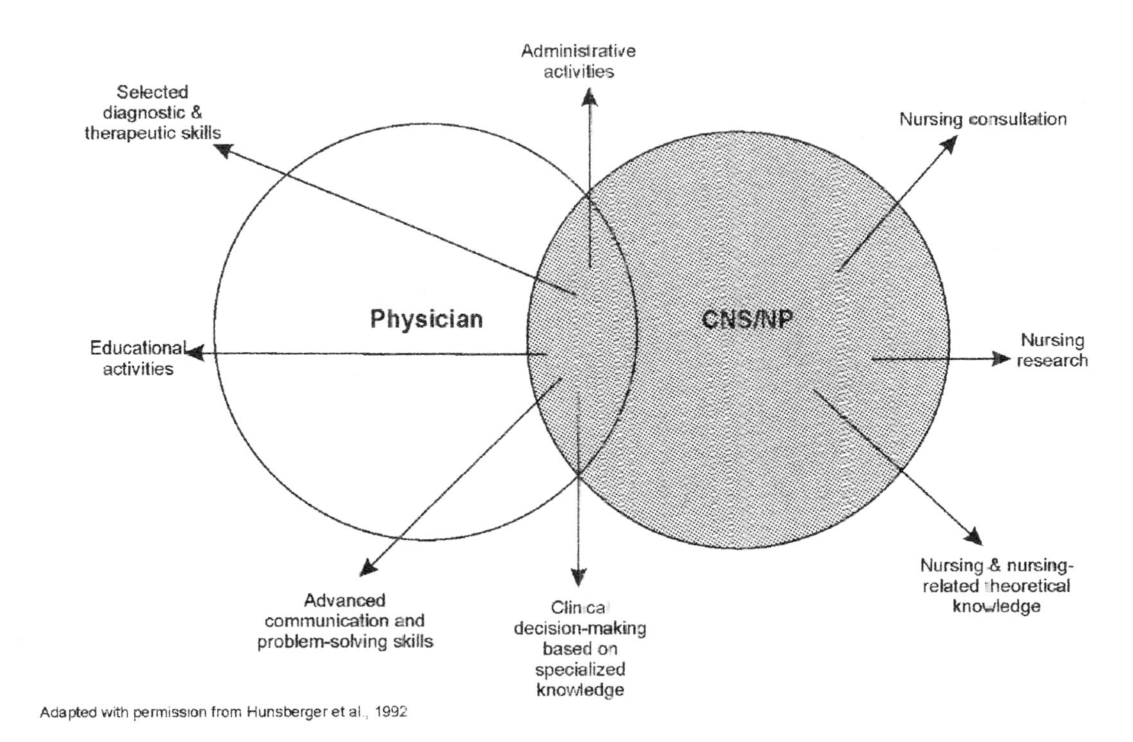

The role of the NP in neonatology was recently evaluated.[55] Graduates from the program were prospectively compared to a cohort of second-year paediatric residents in problem-solving, communication, and clinical skills. Graduating nurse practitioners were evaluated as being equal to paediatric residents on all outcome measures, and the authors concluded that the program was successful in preparing neonatal practitioners for their role. We have also completed a randomized controlled clinical trial, evaluating the care delivered by NPs versus a paediatric resident team. The study demonstrated that the two were comparable with regard to quality of care, parent satisfaction with care, morbidity, mortality, long-term outcomes and patient care costs.[56] The authors recommended that NPs provide appropriate standards of care and should be on a more widespread basis. There has now been widespread acceptance of the role of neonatal NPs in the literature with further demonstration of equal effectiveness with physician assistants and residents in the delivery of paediatric intensive health care.[57-63]

The role of the NP in primary health care is not different from that in the intensive care setting. It is collaborative, "client-centred with a holistic approach that fosters the development of trust between care provider and client."[64] A partnership between the NP and the family practitioner recognizes that each provides a skill and knowledge based on "mutuality of concern for each other as well as for the patient."[65] Way and Jones developed practice guidelines for specific health care functions which help to clarify and formalize direct and indirect consultation between nurse practitioners and physicians in their office-based practice.[64] The success of such a venture in terms of favorable health outcomes for patients receiving NP care was supported by the Burlington randomized trial.[66] In a recent survey, general practitioners in England and Wales were also 90% satisfied with the role of the NP within their practice.[67] However, the function of NPs in this survey was distinctly different from that in the Canadian setting. Ninety percent of respondents expected NPs to undertake tasks such as the measurement of blood pressure, sterilization and maintenance of equipment, the running of health promotion clinics, and the administration of travel immunizations. Less than 40% of the general practitioners felt that nurses were able to diagnose and initiate treatment for certain conditions independently. This again is in sharp contrast to the NP's role in remote communities where they work in isolation, are allowed to perform delegated medical acts, and assume these functions without supervision.

In summary, the nurse practitioner role has changed significantly over time, traversing boundaries into the sacrosanct domain of traditional functions performed by physicians. NPs acquired both clinical and technical expertise to operate in all branches of medicine that span the range from general medical supervision and health maintenance to acute critical care. NPs should be registered to practise in any given setting after proper preparation and an apprenticeship that progresses through stages from direct to proximate to general supervision and, finally, independent function.[51,68]

Acceptability and Conflict in Role Implementation

Site visits to Georgetown University Hospital, Washington, D.C.; Good Samaritan Hospital, Phoenix, Arizona; St. Joseph's Hospital, Denver, Colorado; St. Luke's Hospital (a branch nursery of Children's hospital, Denver, Colorado); and the University of Alberta were used to determine the advantages and conflicts of the neonatal nurse practitioner's role. Similarly, the medical directors and Ontario NICU head nurses were surveyed for their perceptions of the role. The survey was performed before the introduction of the nurse practitioner program and indicated that all the Ontario NICU medical directors and head nurses were in agreement that the NP role should be adopted. It was apparent from the responses that the strength of the role focused on the quality and continuity of patient care with relief of the strained staffing situation. In units with existing NPs, the overall impression supported the fact that they were invaluable team members, used protocols, and consulted with neonatologists to make major decisions. NPs appeared to have an advanced level of independent decision-making on a day-to-day basis and were highly competent in emergency situations. Acceptability of NPs was generally very high with a strong belief that improved, comprehensive patient care derived from their presence. A recent survey of medical staff working with graduates of our NP program indicated 80% of all caregivers felt that NPs had made a significant difference to their level of job satisfaction.[69] NPs were consistent, reliable, provided quality patient care while ensuring continuity with excellent documentation. Their technical expertise and competency made them an invaluable educational resource for nursing, medical staff, and allied health professionals. NPs demonstrated an advanced appreciation of the psychosocial dimensions of neonatology, which made their role in family oriented newborn care exemplary. In my opinion, the most notable comment on the NPs' performance was the recognition that "they guaranteed safe and appropriate standards of care in the NICU." NPs were generally accepted by all professionals with minimal resistance from a few sceptical sectors.

The major reasons identified as being obstructive to the implementation of the NP's role are financial implications, legislation to perform delegated medical acts, level of training and program availability, costs of continuing education, physician resistance, legal restraints, and cost effectiveness.[70] It is not surprising that misperceptions of the role definition and educational preparation of the NP may negatively influence the introduction of the NP in any setting.[71] Traditional programs at the certificate level trained nurse practitioners to undertake a limited number of delegated medical acts and were suited to strictly confined areas of medical care. The scope of practice did not allow for independent decision-making, ordering tests, establishing diagnoses, and prescription of appropriate diagnostic and therapeutic interventions. Practitioner programs, like the one at McMaster, are designed to provide for a broader educational base with specialization occurring during the clinical practicum. Master's degree NP programs in the U.S. currently outnumber certificate programs in a ratio of 3:1, and it has generally been accepted that in the long-term NPs across all specialties should train at the graduate level.[46, 72, 73]

However, a major obstacle to NPs is physician acceptance of equivalency in clinical performance. Physicians are of the firm opinion that the objectives and level of NP educational training is not on par with the medical school curriculum and postgraduate training. Most NPs with master's degree training complete six years of education while a general practitioner has a minimum training of 11 years. In the past, the focus of NP training centred on family-oriented care, health promotion and maintenance. Newer programs teach and rigorously evaluate the theoretical framework of nursing process and advanced practical skills that integrate knowledge from both nursing and medicine.[56,73-75] Moreover, the curriculum content, guidelines for educational preparation, preceptorship, and certification have been standardized to provide internal consistency and credibility to neonatal NP training.[76,77] There is now ample data demonstrating equivalency in practice standards between physician and NPs in defined settings.[10,56,64,66]

In 1993, the American Nurses Association Analysis (ANA) of Studies evaluating NPs in urban locations proved that they provided equivalent or better care than physicians in three major areas: process of care, clinical outcomes, and utilization. The better performance in the areas of quality of care, patient satisfaction and compliance, and on the resolution of pathological conditions, is a reflection of sound training in health assessment, education, promotion, and disease prevention. Physicians continue to argue that the evidence from clinical trials demonstrating the effectiveness of clinical care delivered by NPs is methodologically flawed. The ANA analysis, however, even when restricted to the soundest evidence from only strongest randomized controlled trials, showed no difference or resulted in better outcomes for the NP group.[10,73] Mitchell et al. in their extensive search of the literature also reviewed NP performance in 29 studies in the primary health care setting and 13 in secondary or tertiary level care. They also demonstrated that NPs and physicians delivered similar standards of care, but with improved patient satisfaction and better patient outcomes in defined situations in the NP cohort.[73]

It is not surprising, therefore, that Ontario's policy on NPs focuses on complete autonomy and independent functioning for NPs. This has unfortunately resulted in a major rift between family physicians and NPs instead of encouraging a much-needed, closely-knit, collaborative practice model. NPs can effectively manage 70-80% of industrial health problems and can undertake 90% of the role of the general practitioner.[78-82] They may be more cost effective and sometimes fulfil the role more admirably.

The evidence for cost effectiveness of NP care has never been accurately determined because of the large number of variables involving each study. In the U.S., it has been estimated that $8.75 billion could be saved through the employment of NPs.[83] Similar cost savings could be realized in Ontario with NPs assuming responsibility for well baby care and for delegated primary care services.[80,83-85] However, physicians and physician governing bodies continue to dispute the validity of this data, and legislation in some countries predicates that physicians must retain responsibility for the ultimate welfare of patients and that NPs may only render care under direct supervision.[86,87] Moreover, if these rights are infringed, the medical profession has intervened to bar NPs from clinical practice.[88]

Why are NPs viewed as competitiors rather than collaborators? The main deterrent perhaps stems from financial implications. Jonathan Lomas claims: "NPs remain under-utilized in the health care system because of a perception of oversupply of physicians."[80] The introduction of yet another health care professional into the community, who may provide a service at perhaps a cheaper cost to the health care system, will impact on the numbers of patients currently seen by general practitioners and perhaps on the future supply of physicians in office-based general practice. In the U.S., NPs in primary care can function independently and autonomously and bill appropriately for their services. Medicare, Medicaid, third-party reimbursement by insurance companies, and Federal Employee Health Benefit Plans all provide avenues of income relative to the legislative authority in each state and type of practice.[68,73] This has increased the profile of NPs as individual providers of health care in rural practice, urban centres, and critical care settings. NPs operating independently will vie competitively with primary care physicians on a fee-for-service basis. A fee-for-service form of reimbursement, however, has been viewed as a major disincentive to the employment of NPs in the health care system. The model encourages proliferation of services and health care providers with a corresponding reduction in efficiency.[89] Payment systems based on salary, contract and sessional payments, capitation models, mixed capitations plus limited fee-for-service, or capitation with incentives for collaboration have been recommended.[89-92] The model selected should foster collaboration between NP and physician provider to achieve the most desirable outcomes for the consumers.

Legal and prescriptive authority for advanced nursing practice in the U.S., varies substantially from state to state and has recently been summarized.[93] In Ontario, we were granted approval for the neonatal NP role and the delegated medical acts from the Advisory Committee on Special Procedures of the College of Physicians and Surgeons of Ontario. Committee members were comprised of representatives from the Colleges and Associations of Nursing and Physicians. The introduction of the role in any of the medical sub-specialties such as oncology, paediatrics, cardiac units, or psychiatry will require the same stringent process of approval before implementation.

In my opinion, NPs are the way of the future. In an era of cost containment, public demand for NP services and midwifery practice, and the current success of NPs in community-based primary care centres, secondary, and tertiary care services, strongly advocate the use of NPs as efficient health care providers. In neonatal intensive care, medical staffing difficulties led to a very successful implementation of the NP role.

The need for NPs in neonatal intensive care units across Canada and the States clearly exists, but the number of graduates have been limited by the absence of training centres and financial support for programs, students and graduates.[94]

The scope of NP practice, reimbursement, legislation, and legal accountability are issues that currently undermine integration of NPs into the health care system. Institutions without practising NPs remained sceptical of their scope of practice and had difficulties recognizing how they would integrate into the nursing/medical team concept. The introduction of a new role can be likened to any critical diagnosis in which patients go through the process of denial, anger, bargaining, and depression before final acceptance. We were viewed similarly till the effectiveness of the role was demonstrated.[55,56]

It is futile to ignore the potential contributions of NPs to health care. While encouraging autonomy and independent functioning in the scope of practice, these aspects of the role, in my opinion, are best executed in the primary care setting with a focus on health education, assessment and promotion initiatives, disease prevention, long-term counselling, and management of chronic illnesses. Even in these settings-and more specifically in the complex sub-specialties-a collaborative model between NPs and physicians will provide for highly efficient interdisciplinary function, permit recognition of each individual's knowledge and skills, and will facilitate consultation between care providers. Debate over the demarcation of what is, or is not, nursing or medicine, risks the fragmentation of patient care by dividing members of the health care team at a time when collaboration and increased efficiency in health care delivery is sorely needed and publicly demanded.[6] The optimal goal is consumer satisfaction and safety.

The combined educational strengths and practical skills of the NP/physician team gives clients an access to professionals who can best serve their specific health care needs. The optimum cost-effective mix of NPs, physicians, and allied health care personnel in a given practice setting remains to be determined. The NP role has now received full physician support in specific jurisdictions such as neonatal intensive care. Physicians will soon come to realize that advanced practice nurses are an invaluable asset in their everyday practice. The recent revision of the health reform agenda by the Ontario Ministry of Health has changed emphasis from treatment to disease prevention and health promotion and gives precedence to the integration of NPs within the community.

Chapter Five

Professional Perspective on the Role of the Nurse Practitioner

Kathleen MacMillan

The nursing profession has taken a keen interest in the development of the NP's role and its place in the long-standing struggle for professional identity, education, and autonomous practice in nursing.[1-4,5-7] I believe that the currently proposed model for the generalist nurse practitioner in Ontario actually reflects the preferred role for the registered nurse at the basic level-nursing as it should be practised. For this reason, this discussion of the role of the NP is embedded in the role of nurses in the health care system in general.

Professional Issues that Influence the Nurse Practitioner Initiative

Medicine and nursing are distinct professions that happen to share a small area of overlap in their scopes of practice. This is a critical point from which the definition of the NP's role must be derived, if it is to be viewed as a nursing role and not as that of a medical auxiliary. Medicine is unique among the health professions in that it claims to have knowledge and skills held by other groups having much more education (four year undergraduate degrees) in the field, such as nutrition, nursing, midwifery, and physiotherapy. Medicine is also legislated to perform activities and skills that other health professionals are educated to perform, resulting in overlap with every other professional group.

Historical Perspective

As early as the writings of Florence Nightingale, we have evidence of the overlapping spheres of practice of the two major health professions: medicine and nursing. Nightingale was clear that nursing was a separate, but equal, discipline from that of medicine, and its contribution was unique and complementary to medicine.[8] It is important to note that historical, cultural, and sociological factors (including gender issues) have contributed to the development of nursing as a secondary profession, subordinate to medicine. Nursing is a female-dominated profession which has not been recognized as possessing a separate and distinct professional body of knowledge. The education of nurses has largely been relegated to an apprenticeship model, where, until quite recently, nursing students provided most of the care given in hospitals in exchange for a debatable standard of education.[9] The emphasis on knowledge-based practice and on the use of biostatistics to inform policy and decision-making, which Nightingale brought to the profession,[10] was not incorporated into nursing models of practice until very recently.

While Nightingale has been credited with many of the problems that developed in modern Western nursing's social and professional status,[11] it is more likely that she, too, was limited in what she could accomplish in the mid-nineteenth-century world. Nightingale's model of nursing education has been described as a pragmatic experiment, and the result of enforced compromise by at least one historian.[12] At a time when she might have longed for an equally rigorous education for nurses as for physicians (medicine was just beginning to develop its scientific base), women were not admitted to university in England. Women were admitted to Oxford and Cambridge in 1920, but even then, while they could take all of the courses and write all of the examinations, they could not make a degree bid until a decade later.[13] The nursing profession is still struggling with tremendous social and political opposition to university preparation for registered nurses.

In her historical study of nursing in Winnipeg in the 1920s and 30s, MacPherson stated that nursing was as scientific as medicine was at that time, with nurses studying much of the same basic science content as medical students.[14] Since then, however, while medicine was supported to grow and develop, nursing was largely suppressed and confined.[12] As late as the 1950s, nursing was perceived as subordinate to medicine by doctors, and nursing generally concurred.[15] Since that time, the feminist movement and a general societal rejection of authority have affected the traditional relationship.[15] Later in this century, the distinction between medicine and nursing was vulgarized to the notion that while physicians cured, nurses cared, suggesting that while they might not be as powerful, or as well educated, they could at least be morally superior. The full dimensions of nursing have been better described by Hall (1990) as encompassing all of the components of comprehensive health care: health promotion, illness prevention, care, cure, rehabilitation and support, without undue overemphasis on caring or underemphasis on cure.[16] Nursing and medicine, states Hall, are analogous to two sides of the same coin, and both are needed for the health care coin to have any value. The curative activities that fall in the overlap between nursing and medicine are as much nursing as they are medicine.

An experiment with the implementation of nurse practitioners in Ontario in the 1970s and 80s was only partially successful. The reasons for this are fairly straightforward: there was, and is, no shortage of family physicians in Ontario (although distribution is problematic), no mechanism for reimbursement for NPs' care was created, and legal limitations to the nursing scope of practice resulted in duplication of care with the physician. Any family doctor who wished to have an NP join his or her practice had to supervise and authorize some aspects of care and then pay for the NP's salary out of the global practice income. While this was not exactly an incentive, many NPs did find employment in supportive practices and continue to practise up to the present. All of the NP education programs available in Ontario closed by 1983.[17]

Constraints on Professional Growth and Development

Professional nursing has been prevented from developing and expanding with the development of related scientific knowledge as compared to other professions. This failure to accord nursing with the right to expand as, for example, medicine does with new scientific developments, is a major problem for the profession. It has also contributed to gross under-utilization of nursing knowledge and skill and deprived the public of the therapeutic benefit of nursing as it should be practised.

> "Failure to recognize that nursing is a discrete health discipline allied to but not dependent on medicine has led to the under-development of care as compared to cure and has deprived people, sick and well, of a wide range of therapeutic health services."[16]

The model of the generalist nurse practitioner as it is currently described in Ontario-as 'expanded role nursing' or 'advanced practice nursing'-is problematic for the profession. 'Expanded role nursing' has been interpreted as describing a registered nurse with additional education that permits the nurse to perform medical clinical tasks. Many nurses reject this concept and view advanced practice nursing as encompassing more than just medical tasks.[18] To date, in Canada, there is no professional consensus on a definition of either of these terms. Some of this controversy is captured in debates about the semantic difference between 'advanced practice nursing' and 'advanced nursing practice.' Smith stated:

> ... we are selling ourselves and our current challenges short if we define this core of advanced practice nursing in terms of the medical model, that is, as an expanded knowledge base to support diagnosis, prevention, and treatment of disease.[19]

The term 'advanced nursing practice' is felt to more accurately portray the nursing component of the practice.[20]

Ideally, the role of the generalist nurse practitioner would be that of the basic registered nurse, and the advanced nursing practice [sic] role would be filled by a nurse with a clinical practice focus and graduate education in nursing-a nursing specialist, engaging in the practice of nursing at an advanced level. In both cases, the practice would be clearly within a nursing scope of practice. At this point in time, it would seem that the NP generalist model that is being proposed for Ontario lies somewhere between the registered nurse and the advanced nursing practitioner, although the Nurse Practitioners' Association of Ontario has clearly stated a goal of graduate education for the future.[21] If the question of basic nursing education was settled, a definition of advanced nursing practice preparation would be easier to achieve.

Titles, Roles, and Scopes

The title 'nurse practitioner' is an undesirable one, in that it suggests the NP's scope of practice is different from that of basic nursing, and basic clinical nurses are not 'practitioners' of nursing. The term reinforces the notion that these are nurses who are practising medicine or are 'mini-doctors' because of its links with the term 'family practice physician.'

The nurse practitioner's and the clinical nurse specialist's roles developed quite separately in the U.S. since the 1960s.[22] In some areas, these roles are beginning to merge and alternative models for this marriage are being proposed in the literature.[18] The clinical nurse specialist/nurse practitioner (CNS/NP) model is a controversial one, with many CNSs rejecting the medical tasks and functions that are part of this model, while others embrace them as a way to ensure a role for specialist nursing knowledge in the acute care setting.[22] Certainly, there also is a need for specialist nursing knowledge[23] beyond the acute care setting, but there may be disadvantages to the merger, in the ability of CNSs to meet the needs of the profession, the community and the system, as well as those of the individual client. The current environment tends to reward and reinforce clinical skills related to medicine more than those related to nursing, thus differentially compromising the proportion of time that the CNS/NP might spend in research, education, administration, and practice in nursing. All of these components of professional nursing practice are felt to be important to the CNS's role.[23,24]

The profession is concerned about adding to the nursing scope of practice those aspects which have traditionally been part of medical practice, without also adding to the nursing aspects. Nursing must ensure that we do not merely expand in a medical model-a risk that is implied in trendy terms such as 'extended role nursing,' a term generated by filling a medical gap in service. Such terms tend to emphasize the addition of medical functions to the role and scope of nursing, often to the detriment of the nursing functions. An advanced nursing practice approach to the victim of a sexual assault, for example, would include immediate and long-term counselling of both the victim and family, and support through the legal process beyond providing testimony, in addition to the physical examination, screening, preventive treatment, and evidence collection that describes a traditional medical role.

Currently, the nursing profession is plagued by a plethora of levels, titles, roles, and functions that do not adequately reflect the educational preparation required to fulfil these roles, tend to be task focused, are not legally sanctioned by protection of title or identified scopes of practice, are not transferable across practice settings, and are not meaningful to other health professionals or the public. Furthermore, the roles of the registered nurse (RN) and the registered practical nurse (RPN) have been rendered indistinct by providing opportunities for increased scope of practice for RPNs without providing similar opportunities for RNs and NPs.

The nurse practitioner's role is developing amid this currently fuzzy thinking. Many nurses, let alone those external to the profession, are confused about the difference between the roles of the generalist nurse practitioner, the acute care nurse practitioner, the extended role nurse, the advanced practice nurse, the clinical nurse specialist, and the clinical nurse specialist/nurse practitioner.[25] Added to this, we have nurses in remote areas of the province whose practice is, in some ways, similar to that of the nurse practitioner but who do not have the educational preparation, nor do they use the title. Clearly, there is an urgent need to bring some order to this situation, and the current initiative to reintroduce nurse practitioners to the Ontario health care system is proving to be the catalyst to a vigorous and healthy debate.

Barriers to Implementation of the Nurse Practitioner Role: Socio-cultural Norms

Perhaps the primary barrier to role development lies in socio-cultural norms and values. Here gender issues play a major role in a subtext which includes perception of nurses as 'second best.' The public believes that health care is limited to that care which is provided by doctors, and chiefly in hospitals. Nurses are not perceived as autonomous health care providers, but, as doctors' helpers and hospital employees. There is scant recognition of the many roles that nurses fill outside of the hospital setting, such as home visiting, the community health centre, or the public health department. Few urban Ontarians have had any exposure to the therapeutic value of professional nursing care, in and of itself.

There is almost no recognition of nurses as knowledge workers. Consumers are poorly prepared to accept nurses as primary care providers and may view the NP as a substitute physician or a second-rate provider. The fact that nursing practice overlaps with medicine, and is not dependent on it, is not recognized by the average client; nor is the concept of first-class nursing (nurse as primary provider of nursing care), as opposed to second-class medicine (nurse as provider of medical care in the absence of a physician).

This is not only a consumer problem. Many nurses do not have a perception of their profession that extends to autonomous practice. The phenomenon of professional autonomy in nursing has been correlated with level of education, practice setting, clinical specialty, professional roles, and membership in professional organizations.[26] Eighty-five percent of nurses in Ontario are educated as generalists at the diploma level; the majority practise in acute care settings, and less than 15% belong voluntarily to the professional association.[27] The education of nurses as technical workers designed to provide care for the sick in the hospital setting has contributed to this lack of autonomy. This socialization of nurses has contributed to the existence of a rather anachronistic, pink-collar ghetto. Nurses have been described by at least one nursing leader as "the housewives of the health care system" (D. Hall, personal communication, 1994). Their work is largely invisible, poorly recognized and rewarded, but also essential to the functioning of the organization. The health care system remains one of the last great bastions of the patriarchy.[28]

Reimbursement Models

A second barrier to role development for NPs is financial in nature. The unpaid labour of women has formed the basis for health and illness care for much of history. Nursing as a paid profession has a short history and is still not valued accordingly. The baby boomers are the first generation of nurses who have chosen the profession as a lifelong occupation, instead of a preparation, or a waiting period, for marriage and motherhood. The average nurse is now 42 years of age and, as a mature, experienced professional, has different expectations of professional practice and reimbursement than nurses might have held in the past.

In the past, nursing care was primarily provided in hospitals by nursing nuns and/or by nursing students. The system of education permitted nursing students to become "the exploited drudges of an expanded hospital system."[12] There were few professional nurses in these hospitals, and those who were employed were engaged in educational and supervisory roles, as well as providing the necessary consultation to the novices who provided the direct care. As late as the 1960s, in Toronto, nursing students were counted in hospital ward staffing and provided the bulk of shift nursing care. Outside of the hospital, community nursing care needs drew on the knowledge and expertise of those women who had been trained and educated as nurses, but who no longer worked for wages after marriage. These nurses continued to practise, however, as free health care resources to their communities for the rest of their lives.

As a society, we tend to willingly pay for what we value and can afford. The funding of our health care system, with its emphasis on physician and hospital care, arises from this value system and will require major restructuring if NPs are to become full partners in the system. The fact that NPs failed to gain a place in the health care system two decades ago, largely because of the lack of a reimbursement mechanism, is germane to this initiative.

The role of free enterprise (if any) in a publicly funded health care system is also relevant. Canadian physicians protectively guard their free enterprise status and consistently use their American counterparts as social comparators in evaluating their financial rewards.[29] Difficulties over medical and nursing 'turf' are being driven by economic pressures and competition. The financial base of family medical practice is definitely threatened by the NP's role, and autonomy of practice is probably the greatest friction point.[15]

Legal Restrictions

A third barrier lies in the legal limitations which have been placed on the practice of nursing and on its ongoing development as a profession. Current legislation denies acute care nurse practitioners, and in most provinces primary health care nurse practitioners the ability to practise autonomously in any way which would make it a valid option to physician care or permit nursing to function as a direct access point to the system. Nurses are not able to practise autonomously in the overlap area between medicine and nursing as physicians are. This permits doctors to provide nursing services to the public at doctor prices. In this way, the concept of nursing as a subset of medicine is maintained, and medical professional dominance is assured. In a recently conducted survey of health agencies throughout the province, laws and regulations were seen as a major contributing factor to the limited use of NPs in the practice setting.[30]

One of the challenges of developing the role of nurse practitioners lies in the relative surplus of physicians in Canada. We have sufficient family practice doctors to meet the need for primary illness care. They are not well distributed, however, and many areas of Ontario have been designated 'difficult to serve,' because physicians are not willing to set up practices in these areas. These are not all northern areas-many are in southwestern Ontario. What they have in common is a relatively sparse population that does not support the desired income on a fee-for-service (FFS) basis. In contrast, in many urban centres, we have a surplus of physicians, and we have ceased to derive any benefit from this surplus.

Current Perspective

Today, because university preparation for entry to the nursing profession remains largely an unfulfilled dream, educational preparation for expanded roles within nursing is highly variable and lacks cohesion. Many nurses stubbornly adhere to the notion that nurses do not require a university education as preparation for basic practice. At the same time, clinical nurses are constantly criticized for lacking knowledge and skills that would, for all intents and purposes, require university education in the sciences and humanities to be able to practise competently. Other health professions, such as midwifery, nutrition, physiotherapy, and audiology have had no such difficulty in determining their basic educational preparation.

It is clear today that nursing and medicine do have overlapping scopes of practice. The division between what is nursing and what is medicine within this overlap area appears to be legislatively defined by who gets to practise autonomously and who gets to bill government-insured services to pay for it. In many cases, the discrimination between the two scopes of practice is a geographic one, with nurses practising in a more expanded role in isolated rural or northern areas of the province and strictly limited where access to physicians is greater.

Specific examples of care provided in the overlap area, in which both medicine and nursing are competent to practise, include clinical decision-making related to well baby care, physical assessment, immunization, women's health screening and care, simple episodic illness care or minor injury care, wound care, as well as evaluation of treatment outcomes and drug efficacy or side effect monitoring.[31] For most episodic and uncomplicated chronic illnesses, NPs may also diagnose, order specific screening and diagnostic tests, and prescribe drugs under medical protocol. In many cases, the medical supervision is a token one, consisting of an authorizing signature. In the U.S., NPs have been identified as providing more than 200 coded services that MDs are routinely paid for, with 'infrequent' medical supervision.[32] In all cases, the public is paying physician costs for nursing services, because there is no mechanism to pay for nursing services in our insured health care system.

Critical Overview of the Political Process in Ontario

The political process of implementation of the nurse practitioner in Ontario was unique in many ways. Firstly, unlike the midwifery movement in Ontario, which evolved over ten years and with much public support, the NPs' project was driven from within the profession (the Nurse Practitioners' Association of Ontario / NPAO) and by the Minister of Health, who was a consumer of primary health care by a nurse practitioner. The time frame for implementation was extremely short, taking place over the last eighteen months of the mandate of the New Democratic Party (NDP) government in Ontario. Much of the work was done by a core of committed nurses, on a voluntary basis, through a provincial steering committee and several subcommittees comprised of stakeholders from various nursing groups. These groups included the various nursing bodies: professional, regulatory and labour, and nursing educators and administrators. The subcommittees were charged with examining the various issues related to implementation, such as the placement of NPs, legal and regulatory issues, legislative changes, education and preparation, publicity, and public education.

The Provincial Nursing Co-ordinator, Dr. Dorothy Hall, a retired nurse leader with World Health Organization-based international nursing experience and a track record of nursing project success, was hired by the Ministry of Health to oversee the project. She came to the project with a vision for nursing and a firm belief that the introduction of the NP's role did not represent an expansion of the nursing scope of practice. She viewed it as simply a legitimization of existing practice.

Focus groups that included stakeholders from the public and other related professions were held to examine the issue as broadly as possible. Participants were recruited through various avenues, including consumer groups, community groups, and professional registries. Persons who called the Nursing Coordinator's office with concerns about the NP project were invited to attend. Physicians were well represented in those who were both in favour of, and opposed to, the new role. Physicians who were invited to the focus groups, and declined, in many cases refused to attend when they found that they would not be reimbursed for their time lost from work.

Successes

The major success of the project process can be found in the consensus of the nursing profession and in the wholehearted support for the NP model by most of the major factions. Significantly, all ten of the university faculties of nursing in the province collaborated in the design of a single curriculum that could be shared by all, offered by distance education, and met the needs of both diploma and baccalaureate nurses. The flexible entry required inclusion of a prior learning assessment model and a program which offered degree candidacy for diploma nurses plus the NP certificate (a two-year program), as well as a certificate for nurses who already held a nursing degree (a one-year program). This was done to recognize those nurses in remote areas of the province who were currently functioning as NPs by virtue of their isolation from medical services, and who would likely meet prior learning assessment criteria for knowledge required for the NP's role, as well as to provide access to educational opportunities for diploma-prepared nurses.

Serious reservations about the appropriateness of undergraduate education for NPs were held by at least one university, which was offering a privately funded program for acute care NPs at the graduate level (the CNS/NP model) in response to an identified need in the acute care practice setting. This group clearly viewed the NP's role as advanced nursing practice. The need for a nursing consensus of support was, however, recognized and the faculty participated fully in the final educational plan.

Similarly, the three major nursing organizations (professional, labour, and regulatory) collaborated to support the initiative. While not always in full agreement, the overall need for a unified nursing voice on the NP was recognized and valued by all parties as a necessary ingredient for success. The role played by the Nursing Co-ordinator in achieving this cannot be overestimated and demonstrates the need for the right person in the right place at the right time.

Weaknesses

Early in the process, the Minister of Health decided to use an exemption clause within the *Regulated Health Professions Act* (RHPA) to facilitate rapid implementation of the NP role. The exemption would permit the addition of three controlled acts required for NPs to practise autonomously: communicating a diagnosis, prescribing medications, and the application of forms of energy.[33] This decision was based on the volume of research supporting the safety and efficacy of NPs, a perception that this did not represent an expansion of the nursing scope of practice, and a genuine belief that the public interest was best served by providing the services of autonomous NPs as quickly as possible. This decision turned out to be the Achilles' heel of the project.

Normally, changes in the practice of regulated health professions in Ontario are to be reviewed by the Health Professions Regulatory Advisory Council (HPRAC) and public hearings held. This mechanism was built into the RHPA to permit the expansion of any of the health professionals as need and justification arises. As the time for implementation grew closer, a legal challenge was mounted by the College of Family Practice Physicians and the Ontario Medical Association on the basis of the implementation process-specifically the decision to use the exemption mechanism. The groups involved remained adamant that they were not opposing the concept of NPs; they were merely opposing the process used to introduce the role. The real reason for the legal challenge was more likely related to issues of turf and power.

Subsequently, amid mounting pressure from the medical community, the Minister referred the matter to HPRAC, requesting a rapid response. At subsequent presentations at the HPRAC hearings, the medical objections to the role itself became more explicit. Specifically, doctors objected to nurses communicating a diagnosis and to any form of independent practice.[34] Objections to the educational program's content and length were critiqued on the basis of comparison with medical education, demonstrating that the medical view of the NP's role appears to be limited to that of a physician substitute. This points to weaknesses in the dialogue between nurses and physicians, weaknesses which occurred as much due to socio-political issues as to process issues.

The short time frame for the project contributed to weaknesses in the dialogue between nursing and other professional groups as well. Invitations to participate in focus groups were unsuccessfully extended to other health professionals. Because of lack of response, these focus groups were canceled. It is possible that many of these groups did not have sufficient information about the project, the NP's role, implications for interdisciplinary practice, or enough time to respond. A longer time frame would have provided more opportunity to communicate effectively.

The largely voluntary nature of the human resources available to the project was both a strength and a weakness. The broad range of nursing stakeholders, each with their own vision of the NP's role, made achieving consensus on many points challenging. It also made coordination of various aspects of the project more difficult. Each step taken by each subcommittee required communication, not only across the committees, but across nursing organizations, within the Ministry of Health, and with external stakeholders, to make sure that the various aspects of the project were congruent.

Most of the nursing organizations involved either had little in the way of financial resources or legal restrictions on how their funds could be used, because of their respective mandates. While a participant's travel expenses for attendance at meetings were reimbursed by the government, other expenses were incurred by the nursing organizations or individual nurses in the form of loss of salary. At one point, NPAO approached RNAO for financial assistance (and this was provided), because they were no longer able to bear the unanticipated costs. Participants moved, as the project evolved, between pride and protest about the considerable investment of personal and professional time involved. Current delays in the implementation process due to regulatory issues were causing some nurses to question whether the considerable effort will yield fruit.

Future of the Nurse Practitioner in Ontario

The mandate of the NDP government was ended by an election call without the critical legal issues being resolved. Neither of the other two major political parties expressed strong support for the NP model in their political campaigns; however, the new Minister of Health had indicated that the NPs' educational programs were to proceed as planned. This left the project in some jeopardy, although the HPRAC recommendations supported it. In addition, the vocal support by the medical groups, of the NP model as a concept, while focusing on the implementation strategy as the problem, may have served the NP project well in the long run. If the process issues were dealt with effectively, by pursuing the regular legislative pathways, the basic concept would be more difficult to credibly oppose. It seems that the nursing profession is always held to a different standard of proof of efficacy and safety than other professions, especially when issues of turf and economics predominate.

Three central issues are necessary for successful implementation of all nurse practitioners in Ontario: reimbursement mechanisms, interprofessional relationships, and regulatory support. Firstly, payment mechanisms designed to support the introduction of NPs, and the selection of successful pilot projects are key elements for success. This will depend on carefully selecting initial placement of NPs and on evaluating the outcomes critically. It has been recommended that NPs be reimbursed on a salary basis, and not as fee-for-service (FFS). Support for alternatives to the FFS model for all health professionals has been the position of the professional association for some time.[35] Options for reimbursement for independent NPs' practice, should this occur, are likely to be either salaried or some variation on a capitation model.

The relationship that NPs will have to other disciplines is a major factor to consider. Without the support of a physician colleague, the role will be difficult to implement successfully. There will be the need for referrals for medical assessment and treatment, as well as consultation. Hopefully, referrals will also flow in the other direction from physician to NP, as appropriate. NPs must be included in practice settings in such a way that they are not employees of the physician. An employee-employer relationship makes collegial practice almost impossible and would reinforce traditional doctor-nurse relationships that are not conducive to a collaborative interdisciplinary practice.

Clarification of the respective roles of NPs and family practice physicians (FPPs) is desirable in theory but difficult to achieve in reality. Each professional's practice is likely to be highly individual in nature, dependent on the interests, experience, knowledge and skill of each, as well as on the population served and the context of the practice. Currently, examples of NP/FPP shared practices in Ontario demonstrate a wide range of models of professional relationships and interdisciplinary collaboration.[36]

From a legal perspective, the regulatory support for autonomous practice was acknowledged with the proclamation of the *Expanded Nursing Services for Patients Act* which legally recognizes the role of primary health care NPs in the health care system. The practice of physician initiation and/or review of activities that fall in the overlap area is wasteful of physician and nursing time, costly to the system, and unnecessary. Permitting nurses to independently manage care that falls within the NP's scope of practice is highly desirable and essential to realizing the full benefits of the model.

Attention must be paid to other legislation, for example, the *Public Hospitals Act* (enacted in 1931 and not substantively revised since then), which prevents nurses from admitting and discharging patients from hospitals. An exemption is currently in place to meet the needs of midwives, but a comprehensive review and updating of this Act is needed. Many episodic illnesses that could be treated by NPs might also require short-term admission to hospital for comprehensive general nursing and supportive care. The list of regulatory issues is extensive and requires goodwill and commitment to ensure a positive outcome. Without these supports, the possibility for positive results is limited, and the value of the NP's role curtailed.

Potential Contributions of NPs

There are two possible key contributions of NPs to the health care system. First, the role offers an additional choice of health provider to the public and, second, the NP's role can act as a major catalyst for change in a system which urgently requires reform.

Alternative Provider

As an alternative provider, the NP offers increased choice to the public. As another entry point to the system, the NP offers a nursing approach to primary health care: an approach that is strongly rooted in shared problem solving, empowerment of the client, health promotion, illness prevention, and risk reduction. Such an option also introduces care that meets the needs of the whole person in a safe, cost-effective manner. For example, research findings point to less reliance on pharmaceuticals and improved patient teaching outcomes when nurses provide primary care for the elderly as compared to physicians.[37] NPs also offer an acceptable alternative for primary care of patients with long-term HIV infection.[38] These are just two examples of many populations cited in the literature that could benefit from this category of provider.[39]

Health problems which require the particular knowledge of a medical practitioner will be referred, as will problems that require the services of other health care professionals, such as nutritionists, chiropractors, or social workers.

Catalyst for Change

At its heart, the differing status of nurses and doctors is a quality of care issue and, therefore, an ethical issue.[40] If nursing research findings cannot be put into practice because they must first be approved by the physician, there is a delay in utilization of nursing knowledge that could improve care. The implementation of nursing research findings is often hampered by the current nurse-doctor relationship.[16,41] The introduction of the NP's role could help to change the way in which the public and other providers think of nursing knowledge.

The NP's role offers another opportunity for change. The introduction of another provider, who can provide nursing-based health care services in a less costly and more effective manner, and who is paid in other than a FFS format, is the best hope for fundamental change in the way that health care is funded. It is this fundamental change which must occur if we are to ensure universal access to quality health care services for the public in the future. Such a monumental change will, however, require a powerful push to make it a reality. The introduction of NPs could be this force for change. Offering family practice doctors the opportunity to include a NP in their practice setting, not as an employee, but as a colleague in exchange for an alternative payment mechanism for the practice is one option. The simple fact that the public has an option introduces an element of competition that could induce family practice doctors to critically examine alternative payment structures.

Conclusions

Public acceptance of nurses as primary care providers has other possible dividends. The NP's role will provide an opportunity for the public to experience the full therapeutic benefits of nursing as it should be practised. Acting as a powerful wedge for change, the NP's role could assist in creating opportunities for all nurses to achieve truly professional practice. It also paves the way for other health care professionals to be utilized more effectively. I look forward to the day when we have generalist nurses providing fully autonomous and publicly funded nursing care to clients wherever their services are required, and specialist nurses, with advanced nursing preparation, who provide nursing care to complex and/or specific target populations wherever their services are required. I hope that the term 'nurse practitioner' becomes an historic one-a term that once served us well but is no longer required. I hope that the terms 'extended role nurse' and 'advanced practice nurse' also become extinct, along with such functional terms as 'total parenteral nutrition nurse.' I also hope that nursing takes its rightful place as an equal among the health professions-particularly with its partner, medicine, for neither can truly function without the other. While we are interdependent, it serves neither well if one profession is not permitted to develop and expand and is kept in a permanent state of dependency. I look forward to the day when nursing and medicine-the two great health professions-work as equals to provide the best quality health care by the most appropriate provider, based on findings from mutually collaborative research and practice. I envision a relationship in which both professions recognize and appreciate each others' unique contribution to the health of people.

Chapter Six

Political Implications of Advancing the Nurse Practitioner Role

Susanne Williams

Introduction

Successes in the advancement of the nurse practitioner's role in Canada and the United States have resulted from appropriate influencing of public policy through judicious use of politics. In this chapter, the resurgence of the nurse practitioner's role in Ontario will be used as a case example to analyze reasons for these successes and to suggest what still needs to be accomplished to advance the role more broadly in Ontario and across Canada.

Framework for Analysis

The advancement of the nurse practitioner's role will be discussed within a framework of politics, policy, pressure groups, and political resources. Mason and Leavitt define politics as "influencing allocation of scarce resources ... a process by which one influences the decision of others and exerts control over situations and events."[1] They defined policy as principles or guidelines which govern action. "[Policy] encompasses the choices that a society or organization makes regarding its goals and priorities and how it allocates resources."[1]

The relationship between politics and policy is influenced by several important factors. Policy is shaped by politics. Individuals with special interests seek to influence development of policy by formation of pressure groups. Pressure groups in nursing that have had an impact on the nurse practitioner's initiative in Ontario include the Registered Nurses Association of Ontario (RNAO), the Nurse Practitioners' Association of Ontario (NPAO), the Council of Ontario University Programs in Nursing (COUPN), and the Ontario Nurses Association (ONA).

Pressure groups are more effective if they are organized and possess many and varied political resources.[2] Political resources refer "to anything that can be used to sway the choice of another individual."[3] Presthus has identified two main categories of political resources, socioeconomic and psychopolitical. Socioeconomic resources that groups can possess include a strong financial base, the occupational status ascribed to the professions, a large membership, access to policy makers, legal authority, previous political experience and organizational cohesiveness. Psychopolitical resources include political expertise and efficacy, prestige, public legitimacy, a monopoly of expertise and a collaborative attitude and commitment from its members.[4]

A final element in the discussion framework is the fact that all political resources are tenuous and distributed unevenly.[5] Nursing needs to analyze its effectiveness in capitalizing on the resources it has in comparison to other pressure groups that are using political resources to advance their positions in the nurse practitioner debate. These other organized pressure groups include the Ontario Medical Association and the Ontario College of Family Physicians.

Nursing's Relationship to Politics

The main thesis of this chapter supports the view that the relationship between politics and nursing should be viewed as a good thing. However, from a historic perspective, nursing and politics have not always functioned comfortably together. At best, it might be seen as an uneasy relationship, with many nurses expressing the view that politics is something that is "not done" in the best regulated families.

There have been many barriers to the organized use of politics to advance nursing positions. The greatest barrier is the lack of socialization of women to politics. In the past, because nursing was primarily a female profession, lack of political awareness led to limited knowledge and understanding of the process and art of political influence. In turn, the lack of political expertise has resulted in the profession having impaired access to many political resources, including funding, higher education, experience in the political arena, prestige, legitimacy, and the attention of policy makers.

Within the past ten years, nurses have manifested increasing comfort in their use of the political process. Some of the factors that have influenced nurses' involvement in politics include the feminist movement, the changing status of women in society, and increased education. With these social changes have come improved access to political resources and an increasing political astuteness. Success in the political arena has also served as a positive prototype for further action. A classic example of such a success was the nursing lobby for changes to the *Canada Health Act* in 1984.

With a changing political and economic climate in Canada, the time is ripe for continued improvement in nursing's political success. Severe economic constraints in health, education, and social services; the rise of consumerism; the valuing of choice and improved access by the public; and the decline in consumer and governmental support for traditional professions are all examples of environmental influences which can benefit nursing as it advances the nurse practitioner's role.

Political Implications of Issues Related to Advanced Nursing Practice and the Nurse Practitioner's Role

As yet, there is no agreement among professional organizations, provincially or nationally, on a common definition of advanced practice nursing and its link with specialization, certification, expert practice, and the nurse practitioner's role.[6] As a result, we have a national certification process, without a clear understanding of how to identify nursing specialties and the appropriate educational qualifications. In the debate, many questions arise. These include the following:

- Does advanced practice mean specialization or can a nurse be "advanced" as a generalist?
- What is the difference between advanced practice nursing and advanced nursing practice?
- What are the relationships between expert practice and advanced practice?
- How should advanced practice be regulated?
- Should the education for advanced practice be at the master's level as it is for the most part in the United States?
- What is the relationship between the nurse practitioner role, the clinical nurse specialist role, and advanced practice.[6,7,8]

Others such as Watson ask if it is not time to be clear about the essence of nursing in an advanced nursing practice role, instead of locating the meaning of the role in the scope of medicine.[9]

A lack of national consensus on the nurse practitioner's title, educational qualifications, and role definition has resulted in the role being referred to as expanded practice. What does this mean? How is this conceptually similar to or different from advanced practice nursing? The lack of consensus has resulted in provinces following their own path or "doing their own thing." As an example, in Ontario, the primary health care nurse practitioner is defined as a generalist. The educational qualifications include a post-baccalaureate certificate for nurses who already have a degree in nursing. Nurses prepared at the diploma level are required to take an integrated program that grants them a BScN (Bachelor of Science in Nursing) and a nurse practitioner certificate. However, in Alberta, the proposed title for a practitioner in an expanded role will be 'Community Nurse Practitioner.' The nurse will be a generalist, providing primary health care across the lifespan. The educational qualification for this role is an advanced graduate diploma in community nursing practice.

These differences in titling, education, and possibly role definition contribute to a potential for divisiveness among professional groups across Canada and a lack of comparability with the United States in relation to the nurse practitioner's role. They also have the potential to negatively influence nursing's ability to maximize political resources in a way that will advance the nurse practitioner's role nationally.

Analysis of the Current Success in Ontario from a Political Perspective

While concerns about divisiveness are real, there have been political successes. The resurgence of the nurse practitioner's role in Ontario is a case in point. The key factors in this success were:

- The personal and passionate commitment of the former Minister of Health, Ruth Grier, whose own primary care provider is a nurse practitioner.
- Support from the Minister converged with the New Democratic Party (NDP) government's search for appropriate strategies to address their health reform agenda of cost reduction, increased quality, improved access, and improved consumer choice and satisfaction.
- The Nurse Practitioners' Association of Ontario (NPAO) was well known to the government for its persistent and effective lobbying of the importance and relevance of the role in addressing some of the government's health reform initiatives.
- The effective use by organized nursing groups of some of the political resources identified previously.

While ministerial support and timing were essential, the successful reintroduction of nurse practitioners as part of the Ontario health system would not have been possible without the effective maximization of political resources by the nursing profession.

From the perspective of socioeconomic resources, the key resource and advantage that nursing has is the size of its group. There are over 100,000 nurses in Ontario. During the most recent provincial election campaign, the RNAO pointed out the importance of the size of the group in terms of its electoral potential with the campaign slogan, "one voter in 64 is a nurse."

Over the past few years, nurses as an occupational group were viewed more positively than some of the more traditional professions, such as medicine, in terms of their ability to influence the NDP government. While the support of the Minister of Health was of primary importance, the appointment of Nursing Co-ordinator, Dorothy Hall, who had considerable primary health care and political lobbying experience, improved direct access to the bureaucrats in the Ministry of Health. The establishment of the Joint Provincial Nursing Committee (JPNC), with representation from all professional, regulatory and union groups reporting directly to the Deputy Minister of Health, also provided access to policy makers for discussing issues of importance to nursing, including the nurse practitioner's initiative.

Nursing professional groups were able to maintain their political effectiveness with the new Conservative government after the provincial election in 1995. The appointment of nurse Kathleen MacMillan, as a special assistant in policy in the office of the Minister of Health, strengthened access to key decision-makers and facilitated passage of NP legislation, the *Expanded Nursing Services for Patients Act*.

Nursing also had past experiences to bring to bear on the development of the nurse practitioner project. Experience with previous attempts at initiating the nurse practitioner's role in the 1970s provided a great deal of learning. These previous initiatives also provided a great deal of research data to support arguments for the effectiveness of nurse practitioners.[10]

Adequate finances are seen as a key socioeconomic resource, essential to political effectiveness. Some funds were provided by the Ministry of Health to support the development of the initiative. Without this support, it would have been more difficult for nursing organizations to come together for discussion and agreement.

The effective use of several psychopolitical resources has been identified as influential in the overall process. The collaborative attitude and commitment of nurses and their organizational cohesiveness was very positive. Political expertise gained from the rise and fall of the Ontario nurse practitioner initiative in the 1970s and 1980s contributed to an effective maximization of political resources in this round. As well, organized nursing groups did not take an all or nothing approach to the development of the nurse practitioner's initiative. Nursing, as a whole, demonstrated a willingness to build incrementally in order to effectively re-establish the role, and increase its potential for entrenchment within the health delivery system. Pearson speaks eloquently of the importance of nursing building on incremental successes as a method of long-term political gain.[11]

Political Analysis for Lack of Complete Success in Ontario

While the political resource analysis indicates reasons for success, further critique demonstrates why the initiative has yet to be completed, and why considerable political influence is still needed to consolidate the nurse practitioner's role.

While timing was a crucial factor in the success of the nurse practitioner initiative, it also played a vital role in its lack of consolidation. The NDP government fell before legislation and regulatory changes could be completed to legalize the expanded role functions. As well, because the political resources of nursing were focused on influencing government and capitalizing on the support of the Minister of Health, there was an inadequate amount of time to get the public solidly behind the role.

Nursing exhibited, and continues to exhibit, a lack of adequate political resources. This is especially evident when nursing's psychopolitical resources are compared to those of the main opposing pressure groups, the Ontario Medical Association and the Ontario College of Family Physicians. This reinforces the point made earlier in the chapter that political resources are transient and unevenly distributed.

When socioeconomic resources are considered, the most important impediment to complete success of the initiative is the fact that legal authority for the nurse practitioner's role is not as yet in place for NPs working in acute care. The *Expanded Nursing Services for Patients Act* allows primary health care NPs to function autonomously. However, until all NPs are covered under the Act, there are NPs who will continue to function under medical directives for the 20% of their role which overlaps the scope of practice of medicine, and a key reason for the failure of the nurse practitioner's role in the 1980s will continue to plague this initiative.

While some past political experience was used positively, nurses still demonstrate a naivety of approach and expectation in terms of how things really get done politically. This naivety stems from our historical relationship to politics. Pearson points out how critical it is for nursing to more effectively and deliberately analyze and influence the power structures in political arenas.[11] In this instance, organized nursing probably overestimated the importance of their relationship to the Minister of Health and underestimated the role of Premier Bob Rae in pushing through appropriate regulations prior to the call of the 1995 election.

In relation to the psychopolitical resources of prestige, political expertise, and legitimacy in the eyes of the public, nursing and nurse practitioners come nowhere near possessing the political resource effectiveness of the organized medical groups. Organized medicine has publicly stated that they are not opposed to the nurse practitioner's role per se, but that they did not feel consulted in the development of the process. While they were not consulted broadly, representatives from medicine were invited to participate in nearly all of the planning committees.

Several other factors are reflected in the early opposition of physicians. Under the NDP government, they saw the nurse practitioner initiative as another example of the erosion of their authority within the health delivery system. They had been faced with capping of fees, a change in reimbursement from fee-for-service to salary or capitation, and a decrease in the number of medical school positions. If nursing was more effectively able to maximize psychopolitical resources of prestige, political expertise and legitimacy, nursing would be a stronger counterbalance to the power of medicine. In this instance, medicine might not have been as effective in putting up road blocks to the establishment of autonomous practice for NPs.

Organized medicine has also expressed concerns about the ability of nurse practitioners to function in independent practice (i.e., without direct access to physicians). In general, they believe the nurse practitioner education program does not provide sufficient depth of knowledge and supervised practice to support autonomous diagnostic and prescriptive authority. Concerns have also been expressed about the validity and reliability of research analyses that have been used to support the efficacy of the nurse practitioner's role. Critique has been centred around the use of what they perceive to be outdated American studies.[12]

While they joined the political foray late in the initiative, physicians were effective in mobilizing their political resources. They succeeded in forcing the Minister of Health to refer the pending regulations to the Health Professions Regulatory Advisory Council (HPRAC), an advisory body charged with sorting out jurisdictional disputes between professions. This action substantially meant that these regulations could not be put into effect by ministerial exemption prior to the election.

Is There a Future for Nurse Practitioners in Ontario and Canada?

There is undoubtedly a future for nurse practitioners in Ontario and Canada if nursing continues to learn from political analysis such as this and use their newfound expertise to deal with outstanding issues. In Ontario, there are several issues still requiring attention. As identified above, it is critical that legislative changes be completed to allow for autonomous prescriptive and diagnostic authority for all nurse practitioners. In addition, the rigorously designed evaluation of the entire nurse practitioner's project, including the educational program and client and system outcomes, needs to be completed. To address issues of perceived bias, the research team is multidisciplinary in nature, including nurse and physician researchers and epidemiologists.[13] This research will provide robust, current national data to illustrate the effectiveness of the nurse practitioner's project. A positive evaluation will support the Canadian advancement of the role. If, however, the evaluation does not support the role, then we will have data that identify the changes needed.

Public education regarding the advantages of the nurse practitioner's role within the context of health reform needs to be widely undertaken. This will enhance the development of the nurse practitioner's initiative by capitalizing on grass-root support. The effectiveness of consumer support contributed greatly to the successful establishment of midwifery as a separate, regulated health profession in Ontario.

In conjunction with public education, massive education of the medical community also needs to take place. A positive political action strategy in this case has been to co-opt supporters from within their own ranks. This should continue to include consultation with family practitioners in the design of specific curriculum modules related to diagnoses, use of physicians as preceptors as appropriate, and the participation of physician researchers in the evaluation of the NP's project.

Finally, clarification of mechanisms under which nurse practitioners can be hired and reimbursed within the rubric of health care reform is essential. Unless these issues are addressed, some of the reasons for the failure of the 1980s nurse practitioner's initiative in Ontario will continue to be a problem in the 1990s.

On the national scene, there are several outstanding issues that also need to be addressed. We need to reach a professional consensus and consistency around clarification of definitions for advanced practice nursing, advanced nursing practice, expert nursing, and specialization. National agreement on these issues should also lead to a national credentialing process which will provide clarification of titles. Finally, we need clarity and consistency of educational qualifications for nurse practitioners across all provinces. In the future, it is likely that entry into practice as an NP will be at a master's level. This approach would be consistent with the evolution of the nurse practitioner's role in the United States and rebut some of the arguments that the depth and length of education does not support autonomous diagnostic and prescriptive authority.

In order to deal with the outstanding provincial and national issues, nursing needs to maximize its political resources. Nurses need to learn about their strengths and weaknesses from political analysis of events. Case examples such as the Ontario initiative can be instructive in providing frameworks for such analysis.

One method of maximizing these resources would be the establishment of a strong national association to speak on behalf of the nurse practitioner's philosophy and perspective. It would also assist in identifying issues of common concern and increase NPs' potential for growth by speaking with one voice.

Nurses need to increase their political sophistication, including learning how to influence real sources of power. To accomplish this, the nursing profession needs to do what others of political influence do: financially support politicians who espouse similar values and beliefs, hire lobbyists and political consultants, and develop fund-raising strategies to support political initiatives. Individual nurses need to develop and enhance their knowledge base and capabilities in relation to political action skills. Varying degrees of political expertise are necessary. Not all nurses can run for office. However, the minimum expectation is that all nurses should understand the political process and support nursing colleagues who have the skills and/or legitimate mechanisms to enhance political effectiveness through professional organizations and unions.

Conclusion

As an organized pressure group, nursing has experienced some success in maximizing its political resources in the development of health policy initiatives through the reinstatement of the nurse practitioner's role in Ontario. It is clear upon detailed analysis of the utilization of these resources that nursing still needs to become increasingly sophisticated in the positive use of politics to influence changes within the health delivery system. In order to accomplish these changes, there are implications for individual nurses, professional organizations, and unions. The challenge is ours, but the success will also mean the advancement of the nurse practitioner's role across Canada.

Chapter Seven

The Role of Government in Planning and Implementing the Nurse Practitioner Initiative: Ontario's Experience

Johanne Mousseau & Dorothy C. Hall

The health system in Canada is considered one of the finest in the world. Canadians have been well served by a universal, publicly funded health care system. However, escalating health costs are now threatening the integrity and the principles underpinning our health system. Each province is undergoing tremendous change. There is restructuring in every sector of the health care system; there is devolution of power, in some provinces, to provide regions with the authority and funds to meet the health needs determined by the communities which they serve. Health values are shifting from an emphasis on disease-oriented care to a focus on health promotion and disease prevention and from hospital to community-based services. Appropriate utilization of health human resources is also a major theme in health reform. As a result, provinces are showing a renewed interest in the concept of the NP and in this professional's contribution to Canada's health system.

Historical Overview

Nurse practitioners were introduced into the Canadian health system in the early seventies for the following reasons: to provide primary health services in northern nursing stations because of a physician shortage[1-7] in rural and urban areas,[8,9] and to expand the role of the nurse and other health professionals.[10,11] The nursing community supported the role of the NP, as it believed that nursing's scope of practice was far broader than what nursing was permitted to do. Even then, nursing believed that nurses should perform many of the functions traditionally done by the physician: "...physical assessment, medical history, and some treatments."[12] Nursing leaders, however, did not condone NPs who functioned purely as physician substitutes. The Canadian Medical Association supported the expanded role of the nurse and, with the Canadian Nurses Association (CNA), produced a joint policy statement on the expanded role of the nurse in 1973, in which they envisioned the NP playing a large role in health maintenance.[13,7]

In 1971, the Boudreau Committee was established to examine and define the role of NPs in providing primary care services.[8] It was the Boudreau Report which made the implementation of the NP a high priority in Canada's health care system. The Lalonde Report in 1974 focused on health promotion and disease prevention as approaches to maintaining well-being;[14] this further reinforced the need for nurses working in an expanded role.

The Ontario Council of Health, a senior advisory body to the Minister of Health, submitted a report, advising the Minister about the need for NPs in primary care (the first level of contact in the health care system), "where services can be adequately and safely provided by nurse practitioners, they should not be carried out by physicians."[15] The Council also suggested addressing necessary regulatory changes and remuneration problems. The NP would be paid by salary; however, this would pose problems for most physicians who were on fee-for-service, because they would not be able to bill for those services provided by NPs, resulting in a loss of income.[7,16-18]

Throughout the seventies, studies and discussion papers showed NPs to be safe, accepted by clients, and as effective as physicians.[18-24] The next decade brought a number of reports, promoting primary health care with an emphasis on health promotion, disease prevention, and community-based services.[25-31] In spite of the direction proposed in these documents, NPs were becoming increasingly invisible, compounded by the closure of NP programs in the early 1980s.

In 1984, the passage of the *Canada Health Act* heralded a new era for nursing. Not only were the five principles of Canadian Medicare confirmed (universality, comprehensiveness, accessibility, portability, and public administration), but the door was opened for health care professionals, other than medicine, to provide an access point into the health care system.

The Nurse Practitioners' Association of Ontario continued to lobby political leaders both at the provincial and federal levels. The Association also developed a scope of practice statement and standards of practice for NPs in the early 1990s. The

CNA produced a discussion paper in 1993 which addressed the issues concerning NPs, such as scope of practice, education and research, remuneration, and health human resources planning.[7] The document, produced in anticipation of the revitalization of NPs in the Canadian health care system, warned against governments using NPs as a quick-fix approach to a supply problem in underserviced areas. The question posed by many is whether the NP has finally come of age or is the concept simply a "flash-in-the-pan" again.

Trends in Canadian Health Care Expenditures

Health care expenditures, as a percentage of Canada's Gross Domestic Product (GDP), have risen from 5.5% in 1960 to 10.1%, or $7.2 billion, in 1993.[32,33] Canada is considered to have the highest per capita expenditure on health care than any other country with a publicly funded health care system.[34]

Institutional services account for close to 40% of health care costs, and represent the largest expenditure.[34] An aging population which "...constitute(s) about 10% of the population but use(s) 40% of patient days in hospital,"[34] new technologies in diagnostics and in surgery, increasing service volume and intensity, and rising wage rates[35] have been the major contributors to escalating health care costs. It is interesting to note that the main causes of hospitalizations are chronic diseases, most of which are preventable. An increase in the number of physicians and physician consultations has also had a large impact on health care expenditures.

The escalation of health care costs is not a new phenomenon. In fact, the Ontario Economic Council warned Canadians, as far back as 1976, of an imminent crisis if health care expenditures and costs were not controlled.[36] As health care costs continue to increase, affecting provincial and federal deficits, governments are re-examining the structure of the health system, the focus of health services, and its resources. They are exploring the most cost-effective ways to allocate health care dollars. Health reform and new health initiatives are inevitable. Ontario and Alberta are leading the way in utilizing NPs in their respective health care systems.

Role of Government in Health Care

In the development of health initiatives, government provides the vision, goal, and direction for promoting the health of its people through public policy. Policy formulation is a complex, dynamic process influenced by many stakeholders. Through its policies, government determines who will get what kind of health care, who will provide specific health services, and how providers of health services will be reimbursed. Public, social, and health policies provide direction for health reform. Every health reform and initiative requires policy development and analysis. Different models can be utilized for policy development and analysis. Anderson and his colleagues [37] suggest a systems-based sequential model:

- Stage I (Policy Agenda) involves determining policy issues requiring action by government (e.g., sexual harassment in the workplace).
- Stage II (Policy Formulation) involves identifying relevant options to be developed, considering benefits, costs, etc.
- Stage III (Policy Adoption) involves submitting policy proposals for input by interest groups or stakeholders, before the policy is legitimized through the legislative process.
- Stage IV (Policy Implementation) involves the application of the policy to the issue.
- Stage V (Policy Evaluation) involves evaluating the effectiveness of the policy, using established criteria, and identifying the reason(s) for the success or failure of the policy.

This model fails to identify, in policy decisions, who gets what and the rationale for those decisions; these questions must also be answered in any policy development.

Policy and issue analysis are the most important steps in policy formulation. Dye defines policy analysis as a systematic process which describes and explains the reasons for, and outcomes of, government action and inaction.[38] Stokey and Zeckhauser's framework[39] describes the process for policy analysis, which is often used in policy issue papers.

The steps include:

1. Identifying the context which includes policy problem identification, background information (economic, ethical, political/legal, and social), and stakeholder issues.
2. Identifying policy options which specify policy goals, objectives, and options including a 'do nothing' option.
3. Describing the consequences of each option.
4. Establishing specific criteria to evaluate whether each option meets the policy goals and objectives, and to what extent.
5. Recommending the preferred solution, having considered issues such as effectiveness, protection of the public or human rights, administrative, and political feasibility.

This generic type of framework is often used to develop and analyze policies related to health care reform, including the NP project.

Health Care Reform

With the health care system facing severe financial pressure because of the spiraling costs of high technology, illness care, the fee-for-service system, and reduced transfer payments to the provinces for health, the time is right for health reform and for better utilization of health human resources. The traditional health care system, with its emphasis on physician services and acute care hospital-based services, is being threatened by a variety of social, political, philosophical, and economic forces. These forces also threaten the five principles under which the system operates: universality, accessibility, portability, comprehensiveness, and public administration.[40]

Provinces across Canada have produced health reform agendas designed to ensure more efficient use of scarce resources and to shift the emphasis from treatment to health promotion and disease prevention. Through the reform process, governments intend to find ways to better manage the health care system, invest more in community-based programs, redress long-standing inequities in the system, and take a leadership role in preserving Medicare. Many of the health reforms place new emphasis on health equity, by focusing on groups that have historically faced barriers to access. Other areas emphasized include better management of the health care system, more effective use of human resources, participation and accountability within the system, review of expenditures, redirection of long-term care, and reform of mental health services.

In Ontario, strategies were developed for community health, tobacco use, oncology, diabetic care, and human resources management in health care in the early nineties. Other priorities were identified in the areas of aboriginal health, women's health, children's health, AIDS, and rehabilitation services.[41] The policy framework for long-term care and community-support systems was released in April 1993; the mental health reform document was released in the summer of 1993; the community health framework project is under way, as are rehabilitation, oncology, diabetic care, and hospital restructuring reforms. Long-term care reform and mental health reform will be briefly summarized to provide concrete examples of where NPs could be effectively utilized. Factors contributing to the necessity for long-term care reform include high expenditures for inappropriate or unnecessary treatment for seniors, the need for increased emphasis on social determinants of health, the need to address disease prevention and health promotion, the need to base funds on community needs, increased involvement of consumers in health care, the significant increases in the number of people aged 65 years and older in the next 10 years, and the necessity to reduce expenditures on high-tech acute care. The reform will result in a shift from a medical to a health-oriented service model, from institutional to community and in-home services, from late intervention to early intervention, from an illness-driven system to one that supports health promotion, disease prevention, and rehabilitation services.[42]

Reform in the mental health care system is necessary to address the lack of co-ordination among different services, such as provincial psychiatric hospitals; general and specialty hospitals; community mental health programs and health services funded on a fee-for-service basis; the high proportion of funding spent on hospital-based mental health services; the difficulty linking with appropriate community-based services after discharge from the hospital; and the shortage of case management, crisis intervention, housing, and other support services.[43]

One implication of health care reform for the NP's role relates to the priority set by provinces to ensure better utilization of our current health human resources and to ensure that planning results in the most cost-effective and appropriate providers. The impact of reform on NPs is raised in the Barer-Stoddart Report [44] and the Ontario Goals and Strategic Priorities.[41]

Barer-Stoddart Report

In March 1990, the federal, provincial, and territorial Deputy Ministers of Health requested a discussion paper on physician resources. The report, prepared by Professors Morris Barer and Greg Stoddart, was submitted to the Deputy Ministers in July 1991. While the Barer-Stoddart Report,[44] as it has come to be known, addresses physician resources, the authors' identification and discussion of relevant issues and recommendations have significant implications for the NP's role in Ontario. Some of the issues relevant to NP utilization follow.

In 1964, the population served per (active civilian) physician (including interns and residents) in Canada was approximately 775. It has steadily fallen to approximately 455.45 The growth rate in the number of active civilian physicians has exceeded the rate of population growth each year for almost 40 consecutive years, starting in 1952. The costs to educate the additional physicians, and the fee-for-service reimbursement system have contributed to increased health care costs. Barer and Stoddart identified this unjustified rate of growth as a problem, and attribute it to an excessive undergraduate enrolment in medicine and a lack of control over the international medical graduates (IMGs) entering practice in Canada.

All provinces have relied on IMGs to work in rural and sparsely populated areas, which are less attractive to most Canadian-trained physicians; however, the number of IMGs adds significantly to the physician supply in the country. Barer and Stoddart recommended a reduction of approximately 10% in current domestic entry class size, and a reduction of Canadian reliance on IMGs in the longer term. Key informants suggested to Barer and Stoddart that an emphasis be placed on ascertaining areas of clinical work where physicians are not necessary for the provision of medical services in order to guide decisions on physician supply.

Another problem identified by Barer and Stoddart was the imbalance between the number and mix of residency training positions and the population need. According to the report, both the number and mix of residents are driven by the need to provide clinical service, often around the clock and at low cost. This situation requires long hours of clinical service by residents that result, at times, in care of suspect quality and also in reduced ability to secure educational value from clinical exposures.

Barer and Stoddart recommended that the national capacity for residency training be determined by the educational needs of graduates of Canadian medical schools, not by clinical service imperatives. Consequently, they recommended a 10% reduction in the overall numbers of residency training positions funded by provincial ministries of health.

Barer and Stoddart identified significant geographic variation in physician supply. This means that necessary services are not available to some Canadians in a timely way without substantial inconvenience, and that some regions have more physicians than are required to meet the medical care needs of the population.

Throughout their document, Barer and Stoddart made a number of recommendations related to the use of non-physician personnel in the delivery of care. Barer and Stoddart explained that compelling evidence has accumulated suggesting significant potential for the deployment of personnel with education different from physicians in certain areas of medical delivery where equal competence has been demonstrated. NPs, psychologists, social workers, physiotherapists, and family counsellors all represent potentially significant, but largely untapped, substitution potential. They recommended that establishment of new training programs, for extended duty nurses and other personnel able to provide some of the services traditionally provided by physicians, would seem appropriate in light of their recommendations for reductions in the numbers of physicians trained and entering practice in Canada. The development, location, and funding of such programs should be considered key components of a new national physician resources strategic policy package.

Stoddart and Barer point out that there is considerable overlap in the training of health professionals. While this in itself is not a problem, the difficulty is that virtually everything covered in medical education becomes 'medical practice' and, therefore, the exclusive domain of licensed medical practitioners.

This monopoly of clinical activity by the dominant profession has important implications for other policy areas. First, physician supply is affected because estimates of the need for physicians will, by definition and assumption, be overestimated relative to the requirements implied by having physicians provide the services only they are trained to provide. Second, expenditures on medical care are likely higher than necessary because differently educated personnel are restricted from performing some tasks. Third, the geographic maldistribution of physicians might be less of a problem if, for example, NPs were more widely available.

Stoddart and Barer recommended the elimination of exclusive fields of practice and their replacement by a more circumscribed set of exclusive acts and reserved titles to address overlapping scopes of capability of physicians and other health care personnel.[46] They note:

> ... scientific evidence on, and practical experience in the [cost] effectiveness of nurse practitioners have not been translated into regulatory reform. It is ironic that the scope of practice for physician extenders and substitutes is in reality very elastic-expanding when physicians are not available, contracting when they are.[46]

Included in their discussion regarding residency training, Barer and Stoddart recommended that clinical services now provided by residents, but which are not essential for their specialty training, should be provided by other health care personnel. The most commonly heard suggestion from their interviewees was that expanded duty nurses and physician assistants be trained to assume these clinical roles. The Ontario Council of Administrators of Teaching Hospitals (OCATH) and the Council of Ontario Faculties of Medicine (COFM) Committee on Alternatives to Residents for Patient Care discouraged the introduction of physician assistants into the health care system because there was concern that another layer of health care providers would increase fragmentation of care.[47]

With respect to geographic maldistribution, the solution most often mentioned by those interviewed for the Barer-Stoddart Report was the development of new training programs for alternative health care personnel. Receiving particular mention were programs for NPs, extended duty nurses, and physician assistants. A number of interviewees emphasized that care must be taken to ensure Canada does not simply repeat the failure with NPs in the 1980s, by ensuring that the organizational, financial, and regulatory environments do not discourage the use of these practitioners once they are trained.

Those interviewed for the report suggested that more use be made of community health organization-type models and that more emphasis be placed on developing clinical teams to deliver services to replace physician-dominated models of care delivery. They suggested that medical advisory boards in hospitals should be replaced by professional advisory boards that encourage teamwork and eliminate professional domination by physicians. They also noted that more nurse specialists be trained.

Government Initiatives Related to Physician Numbers

In 1993, Barer and Stoddart reported that provincial Ministers of Health planned to implement a phased reduction of 10% in the number of funded residency training positions. However, they noted that the "necessary complementary initiatives in the areas of residency service replacement, foreign medical graduates, and complementary and substitute personnel training are lacking."[46]

Historically, the Ontario Ministry of Health has supported the creation of residency service replacement by NPs. In 1983, it funded a pilot project to study the need for clinical nurse specialists/neonatal practitioners (CNS/NPs) to fill the service requirements created by cutbacks in the number of paediatric residents in tertiary level neonatal intensive care units (NICUs). Since 1983, funding has permitted a needs assessment for CNS/NPs, definition of the CNS/NP role, development and evaluation of an educational program to train CNS/NPs at the graduate level, and implementation of a randomized controlled trial to compare the effectiveness of CNS/NPs with paediatric residents in the care of neonates in a tertiary level NICU.

From 1983 to 1990, the number of paediatric resident positions declined by 17%.[48,49] As a result, advanced practice nurses (CNS/NPs) assumed many of the service responsibilities traditionally performed by residents. With the introduction of CNS/NPs into NICUs in Ontario, the paediatric resident requirement could now be based on educational objectives rather than on service needs. As the ministry implements further reductions in resident training positions, it is likely that the CNS/NP model can be applied to numerous other secondary and tertiary health care settings that have traditionally relied on residents for patient care.

Although numerous studies have repeatedly shown that 50-90% of activities performed by physicians can be done by NPs, maintaining a high quality of care at a lower cost, there is a justifiable reluctance to add new health providers to the system in Ontario. One main reason is a rich supply of general practitioners and family physicians; in fact, NPs have flourished in areas where there are few physicians. The formal introduction of NPs into the system can be financially feasible only if it is accompanied by a reduction in the number of physicians and/or a change in physicians' reimbursement structure to reduce the current expenditures. Otherwise, physicians could still drive the fee-for-service system to maintain the demand, while at the same time the ministry would incur additional salary costs for NPs. Given the ministry's recent steps to control the number of physicians in Ontario and the priorities of the health reform agenda, the time is right to maximize the use of NPs.

Ontario's Goals and Strategic Priorities Working Document

A consistent thread throughout the Goals and Strategic Priorities[41] document in Ontario is the focus on prevention, health promotion, and community-based care. These themes surface in similar documents in other provinces.

The Ministry of Health plans to address the need to enhance community-based primary health care in Ontario with an emphasis on health promotion and disease prevention through primary health care reform. With the reallocation of funding from the illness treatment sector to the promotion of health and disease prevention, structural reorganization of the delivery system has resulted in the funding of an increased number of community health centres (CHCs) in Ontario. Well-functioning CHCs are based on group medical practice, effective use of non-physicians, particularly nurses, consumer/community participation in governance, non-fee-for-service payment for medical services, and a focus on health promotion and disease prevention.[50]

NPs have the qualifications to fit the needs of community directed health services. Provision of primary health care by NPs fully utilizes nursing knowledge and expertise about wellness care, family-centred care and communication skills, and provides an effective option to meet the needs of the public. CHCs currently in operation in Ontario rely heavily on NPs in the delivery of primary health care. If the number of CHCs in Ontario increases, so will the demand for NPs.

Primary Health Care Reform

Another initiative now under way at the Ontario Ministry of Health is primary health care reform, which is intended to address issues of access, quality and continuity of health care. The NP initiative is linked to this strategy because of the NP being a primary health care provider. Decisions concerning health human resources planning cannot occur without having addressed the direction of primary health care, delivery models, system integration, and coordination. Opportunities for NPs will emerge with the development of the primary health care delivery models, and with the creation of a coordinated primary health services system.

Hospital and Community-based Emergency Health Care

Review of hospital and community-based emergency health care is a very important aspect of hospital redirection in Ontario, especially in small and rural communities. Both the Scott [51] and Rourke[52] reports express a sense of urgency in dealing with some of the critical problems associated with delivering emergency health services in these communities. Nursing's role is integral to good, accessible emergency services. Certainly NPs could play a significant role in triaging, in assessing and managing episodic problems, and in providing 24-hour coverage with physicians and other health professionals.

Mental Health Reform

In 1993, the Ontario Ministry of Health announced a ten-year strategy for reforming the province's mental health system. The new system places increased emphasis on health promotion, disease prevention, and community-based programs, using hospitalization only when clinically necessary. It improves access to services, tailors services to needs, provides community and informal supports to clients and their families, and provides services that are sensitive to gender, culture and race, and that meet the needs of underserved populations (women, aboriginal peoples, members of ethnocultural groups, francophones, youth, the elderly, and people with more than one diagnosis).

Over the ten-year period, the proportion of the mental health budget spent on institutional care, excluding fee-for-service expenditures, is expected to drop from 80% to 40%, while the proportion spent on community services will increase from 20% to 60%.[43]

In the reformed mental health care system, NPs could play a major role in the provision of community-based prevention and health promotion services, in counselling for emotional and relationship problems, in providing inpatient and outpatient care to people with chronic mental illnesses, in providing client and family support, and in working with disadvantaged populations. As with other reforms, the emphasis is on de-institutionalization, consumer and family awareness and active participation in health care, and appropriate use of health care workers in institutional and community services.

Long-Term Care Reform

In reforming the long-term care sector in Ontario, NPs could play an increasingly active role in certain levels of curative care, health promotion, disease prevention, and wellness counselling of the increasing population over 65. Much of the care recommended in the reform deviates from the traditional m ical model. The focus is on the maintenance of existing health and on episodic care for a variety of debilitating conditions. The focus of care is one that encourages de-institutionalization, less reliance on pharmaceuticals, consumer awareness, and active participation in one's health care. It requires the integration of health and social services, and appropriate use of health care workers in the community.

Implementation of the long-term care redirection will depend upon a number of agencies in the communities. These agencies can work with NPs in public health departments, in home nursing agencies, and/or in CHCs. NPs can act as primary caregivers and coordinators of the client's care in the community in collaboration with the family physician. The NP can assess and diagnose clients and plan, manage, and coordinate care as required. The NP can also be utilized in long-term care institutions providing similar services and managing long-term problems, such as incontinence and cognitive impairment.

In provinces across Canada, the health care reform agenda increases the focus on prevention, health promotion, and community-based care within the context of effectiveness and economic efficiency, and prompts an examination of traditional delivery of health care. Increased utilization of NPs in all settings of health care delivery is consistent with the provinces' reform agendas.

Health Human Resources Strategy

As part of health care reform, governments have been searching for ways to provide more comprehensive and effective primary health care. Restructuring of the health care system cannot occur without attention to its human resources. In assessing the strengths and weaknesses of the existing health care system and its resources, the Ontario Ministry of Health realized that the system had failed to make the best possible use of registered nurses and their knowledge and skills, and to encourage the development and use of new nursing knowledge. To ensure that the public had the full therapeutic benefit of nursing, the ministry began to look again at the role of the nurse practitioner. In 1993, a series of nursing roundtables were held to address issues such as the role nursing can play in health reform and better utilization of nurses in Ontario's health care system.

In 1993, the Provincial Co-ordinating Committee on Community and Academic Health Science Centres Relations (PCCCAR) met to discuss issues of mutual concern to district health councils and academic health science centres. Issues of concern included the medical postgraduate training system and issues related to health human resources planning for physicians. One of its subcommittees-the Subcommittee on Underserviced Area Needs-developed a strategy, outlining principles and a framework for health human resources planning for physicians in Ontario, to address the needs of underserviced and all other areas of the province.[53] Although PCCCAR and its subcommittees have focused on physicians to date, other health care providers are included in their recommendations. The PCCCAR reports will provide the direction for health human resources planning in Ontario.

The goal, in health human resources planning, is "to achieve the most effective, flexible and cost-efficient use of our [province's] key asset, people, in order to realize Ontario's vision of health."[31] The Ministry is presently developing a comprehensive provincial human resources strategy, based on population needs and linked to a national plan. In terms of physician resource management, some initiatives are addressing the entry of IMGs into the Ontario practice pool and medical school enrollment. The implementation of the Pools Framework for postgraduate training has limited the number of IMGs trained annually to 24.[54] In September 1993, Ontario began reducing medical school enrollment; the University of Toronto reduced its enrollment from 252 to 177.[54] Other reductions are in progress.

Health human resources management includes the planning of nursing resources. With health care restructuring and changing health needs of the population, many nurses find themselves unemployed and having to update their knowledge and skills to meet the needs of the population and the work setting. The Ministry of Health is working with the Ministry of Education and Training to ensure that the educational preparation of nurses is guided by the health needs of the population. Furthermore, the Ministry is beginning to examine, with nursing stakeholders, the number, mix, and distribution of nurses in Ontario, which will surely have an impact on enrollment in nursing schools. Finally, the NP project, a health human resources management initiative, is being integrated into other planning activities related to other health strategies. This dovetails with strategies regarding primary health care and hospital and community-based emergency health care.

The Ontario Ministry of Health has started with the NP working in primary care settings, in particular the community, providing primary health care. The next step is to address the need for NPs and Clinical Nurse Specialists (CNSs) in specialized areas of the acute care system.

Planning and Implementing the NP Initiative

It is important to note that the role of the NP is not new to Canada; NPs have been working primarily in remote areas of most provinces. In Ontario, about 250 nurse practitioners work in rural and urban areas. Some work in multidisciplinary teams and some in settings where there is no physician or other trained health care provider. Most NPs work in primary care settings. The proposed plan to educate and employ NPs recognizes and legitimizes the role that these nurses are now playing in health care. It does not create a new role.

In February 1993, to assess the potential for nurse practitioners in Ontario, the Ministry of Health asked McMaster University to prepare a discussion paper on nurse practitioners. McMaster's paper, Utilization of Nurse Practitioners in Ontario,[55] was released in the fall of 1993. It reviewed the history of NP education and employment in Ontario. The report emphasized the safety and effectiveness of service provided by NPs, noted the high level of public acceptance of NPs, and recommended that NPs be used more widely-particularly in primary health care. Effective utilization of NPs is presently compromised by an oversupply of physicians (especially in urban areas), lack of career opportunities, lack of appropriate remuneration mechanisms, and attitudinal barriers on the part of some physicians.[56]

The NP Project: A Five-Step Process

In November 1993, the Ontario Minister of Health asked Dorothy C. Hall, the ministry's Nursing Co-ordinator to plan and manage a project to reintroduce NPs into Ontario health services. The NP project consisted of five steps:

Step 1: Prepare a position paper that provides a clear statement of the role of the NP and outlines the concept and principles that would be the basis for a workable plan to educate and employ NPs.

Step 2: Prepare a detailed plan for the education and employment of NPs in Ontario.

Step 3: Organize and conduct focus groups with key stakeholders in the health care system to identify barriers to implementing the plan and strategies to overcome barriers.

Step 4: Implement the plan promptly and effectively.

Step 5: Evaluate the project and monitor its progress.

The Position Paper

The office of the Nursing Co-ordinator prepared a draft position paper[57] which was reviewed and revised by the province's nursing regulatory body, professional nursing associations, McMaster University, and the Ministries of Health, and Education and Training. The paper outlined the concepts and principles for developing tho plan for the education and employment of NPs. The principles emphasized that nursing is a fundamental human activity and a discrete health discipline allied to, but separate from, medicine. The paper further reinforced that nursing in and of itself is therapeutic, and the failure to make full use of the knowledge and skills of registered nurses has denied the public many of the therapeutic benefits of nursing.

Model for the Planning and Implementation of NPs

Dorothy C. Hall designed a planning and implementation model[58] to guide the Ministry's Steering Committee and five subcommittees. Issues of education and evaluation, laws and regulations, placement and service patterns, fiscal considerations, and publicity and public relations are specific components of the model. These are the crucial elements to successful implementation of the NP's role. All five components of the model are weighted equally in terms of importance and are interdependent. (Fig 5) Education and evaluation cannot be developed without consideration of the other components. Each aspect of the model also addresses the barriers to full utilization of the NP's scope of practice. From the beginning, the model has been nursing-oriented despite the focus on medical functions related to the needed regulatory changes.

The aforementioned components were addressed by the subcommittees, which fed their information back to the Steering Committee, which made the final recommendations in its report.[59] The committees included representation from Ontario's regulatory body for nursing, nursing associations, the nursing union, university and college schools of nursing, institutional and community nursing services, the medical profession, and the Ministries of Health, and Education and Training. The reports from these committees formed the plan for educating and employing NPs in Ontario. In the process of preparing the plan, the Steering Committee identified the importance of an assessment of the need for NPs in Ontario.

Needs Assessment

The Ontario Ministry of Health commissioned McMaster University's School of Nursing to assess the need for NPs in Ontario. The study, completed in September 1994, addressed the current and future need for NPs, the role of NPs in providing primary health care, barriers to implementing or expanding the NP's role, present and future supply of NPs, future need for NPs, and unmet needs in underserviced areas. The needs assessment utilized four major sources of data: primary care agencies in Ontario; the province's Registered Nurses (RNs), including presently practising and non- practising NPs and Registered Practical Nurses (RPNs); health care planning bodies in Ontario; and existing data from the Ministry of Health.

Figure 5
Nurse Practitioner Implementation Model
Ontario Ministry of Health Nurse Practitioner Initiative

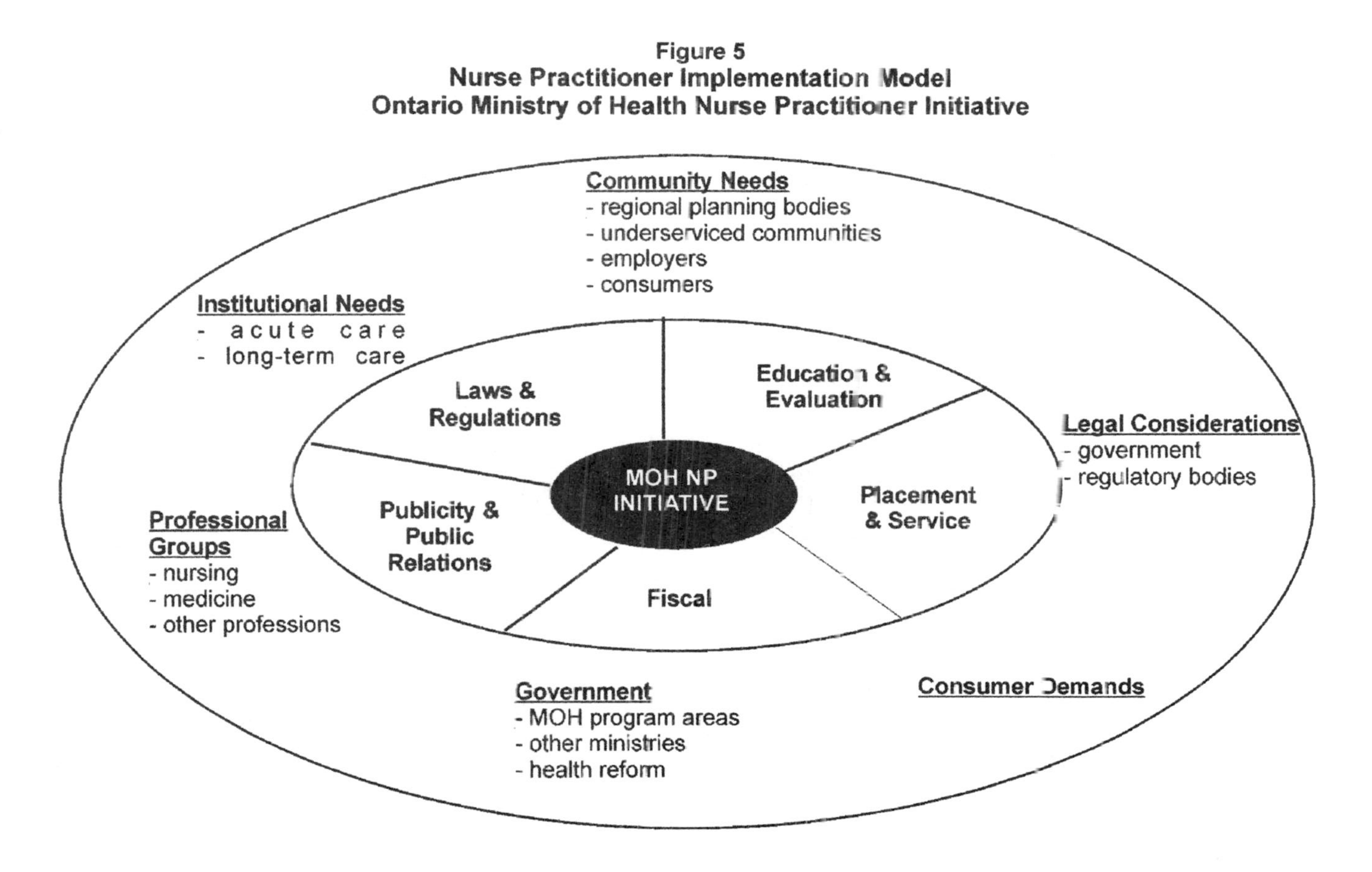

Responding primary health care agencies indicated a need for 996 NPs, particularly for emergency rooms, home health services, and long-term care facilities.[56] (This projection may be higher if non-respondents are considered.) The needs assessment provided valuable data for health human resources planning, including barriers to NPs fully functioning within their scope of practice and barriers to implementing the NP's role.

The major reasons cited for NPs not currently performing the clinical activities which they should be performing were that NPs were not included in the current practice pattern, lack of formal education (and continuing education) programs for NPs, lack of availability of NPs, lack of enabling legislation, lack of funds, and physician resistance. Furthermore, the four most frequently identified barriers to implementing the NP's role included: unavailability of qualified NPs, lack of legislation to enable NPs to perform clinical activities traditionally performed by physicians, reimbursement of NPs, and unavailability of continuing education for NPs.[56] The needs assessment reinforces the importance of addressing the barriers which have prevented NPs from being fully utilized.

Focus Groups

In the summer of 1994, the Ministry of Health held focus groups to assess the strengths, weaknesses, opportunities, and threats related to the implementation of NPs. Participants were also asked to develop strategies to overcome the barriers, and therefore, ensure that NPs were integrated into the system and used effectively. Five groups of stakeholders were identified: district health councils, consumers, the nursing profession, medical and dental professionals, and allied health professionals. The latter group did not meet due to poor response. Instead, a fifth focus group, consisting of community health centres, community hospitals, and other agencies, was selected as a result of discussion in other focus groups, concerning employment issues.

Focus groups provided interesting and valuable feedback and recommended the following:

- the role and scope of practice of the NP be defined clearly and in detail;
- the role and scope of practice of other primary health care providers, including other nursing professionals be defined clearly and in detail;
- any overlap in role and scope, as well as the differences between the professionals, be clearly laid out and explained;
- the ways in which primary health care providers will work together be explored and assessed;
- information about the various roles, scope of practice, and working relationships be communicated clearly to the public and other professionals;
- systematic changes be made to support the defined roles, including regulatory changes, titles, registration process, education programs, funding systems, and other incentives;
- the final program be carefully evaluated to ensure that it is providing the anticipated benefits of improved patient outcomes, cost-effective care, and stronger partner-ships/ relationships in the primary health care system; and,
- that all this be done in consultation with the stakehold-ers in the system and those with the ability to influence the system.[60]

These recommendations mirror those made by the members of the Ministry's NP Steering Committee. The regulatory body for nursing has done much of the work related to the NP's scope of practice. The education sector and the government are now addressing the other recommendations.

Education of NPs

The academic preparation of NPs must include the knowledge and skills necessary for more complex independent clinical decision-making related to the broad scope of practice in primary health care. Although there is a move to graduate-level preparation of NPs in the United States, governments in Canada support baccalaureate-prepared NPs. Alberta has recently made that decision. The Ontario Ministry of Health approved a post-baccalaureate program for NPs, recognizing that primary health care is a complex entity as it encompasses many aspects of care. In fact, the government of Ontario requested that the following requirements be met by the university schools of nursing involved in the education of NPs:

- that the educational programs provide the advanced knowledge and skills needed by RNs to practise safely and effectively as nurse practitioners;

- that all registered nurses, regardless of their basic nursing education, have equal opportunity to enter the program;

- that the program be flexible enough to meet nurses' needs;

- that the educational program be accessible to registered nurses in the province, including those working in remote areas, and to francophone nurses;

- that all NP students receive the same knowledge and skills, regardless of where the educational program is offered;

- that the needs for continuing education for NPs be addressed; and

- that the NP education program meet the needs of aboriginal people.

The ten university schools of nursing, offering the program, worked together and created a unique program meeting the requirements set by the government. This program, funded for five years, began in September 1995. The Ministry of Education and Training (MET), which has been actively involved in the planning phase of the project, will consider future funding of the NP program, following an evaluation process. The program already meets most of the criteria used for new program funding approval.

Laws and Regulations Governing NPs in Ontario

Registered nurses in Canada are governed by the various provincial nursing statutes which describe their scope practice. Regulations spell out, in detail, what registered nurses can do within the meaning of the statute(s). In the settings where they provide care, nurses may also be governed by a number of other laws and regulations. To ensure that nurse practitioners make full use of their knowledge and skills and carry out the role assigned to them, there are statutory and regulatory changes which must be made. In Ontario, these changes include revisions to the *Nursing Act*, 1991, to include the three extra controlled acts.

In providing care, NPs may also be governed or affected by other related legislation. In Ontario, these other statutes may include, for example, the *Healing Arts Radiation Protection Act* to prescribe x-rays, the *Laboratory and Specimen Collection Centre Licensing Act* to order laboratory tests, and the *Narcotics Act* to prescribe some narcotics. Narcotic legislation is controlled federally; therefore, the Federal Minister of Health would need to change the *Narcotics Act*. This would require negotiation between the province and the federal government.

Whether they are working as part of a multidisciplinary team or working in isolated settings with no other health professional, NPs must have the authority to refer clients to and consult with other providers. RNs who are practising as NPs do not presently have the authority to refer clients to medical specialists or to other services in the health care system and have these services covered by health insurance. To ensure that nurse practitioners are equal partners in health care delivery and are able to refer clients, nursing and medicine must work together to assist government in developing appropriate corporate policies or necessary regulatory changes regarding medical referrals made by NPs.

In proposing the necessary legislative and regulatory changes, a number of steps needed consideration:

- the definition and description of the role and scope practice of NPs by the regulatory body (CNO) with input from professional nursing associations;

- the appropriateness and need for NPs performing proposed controlled acts (assessed through meetings with key stakeholders);

- extensive legal consultations regarding the NP's scope of practice, in particular the area of practice shared by both nursing and medicine, and the approaches used for making legislative/regulatory changes;

- advisory committees, consisting of experts in nursing, medicine, radiology and pharmacy, to provide the Ministry with advice regarding areas such as diagnosis, prescriptive authority, and authority to order laboratory, diagnostic, and screening tests;

- meetings between the regulatory body, government, and other key stakeholders to further qualify or delimit the controlled acts, if necessary;

- policy approval of the proposed legislative and regulatory changes, including the content of the regulations at senior levels of the Ministry of Health; and,

- passage of the legislation.

In Ontario, there are two ways to change the provincial legislation that defines nursing practice. The first is to change existing legislation and regulations by amendments to the *Nursing Act,* 1991, *the Regulated Health Professions Act,* 1993 and other relevant statutes. However, the proposed amendments would be debated through the legislative process and, with the government's full legislative agenda, it could take a long time to make the needed changes. The use of an exemption regulation under the RHPA is the other route whereby changes regarding controlled acts can be made quickly without going through the legislative process. This is not perceived to be the best route for changing legislation regarding a profession's expanded scope of practice. The government referred the proposed expanded scope of practice for NPs to the Health Professions Regulatory Advisory Council (HPRAC) for advice in February 1995. The HPRAC report on NPs was released in June 1996, after three rounds of consultations with key stakeholders, recommending an expanded scope of practice for NPs through proposed legislative and regulatory changes.

Placement and Service Patterns

Nurse practitioners are only one of a number of health can providers. If NPs are to be an effective part of the health system, their employment should be looked at as part of a broader health human resources planning strategy. Placement of NPs began with the needs assessment and discussion with different government program areas in health. As a result, NP's have been represented on working groups which are designing and planning service delivery models, such as models for primary health care; therefore, NPs are involved at the decision-making level.

To ensure that NP services are integrated successfully with those provided by other practitioners, NPs would initially be placed within appropriate existing organizations and agencies, such as community health centres (CHCs) and health services organizations (HSOs). When there are no appropriate organizations and agencies in an underserviced community, the government might work with a regional planning body, for example, to develop a process for establishing NP practices which could serve underserviced communities. With their knowledge and skills in comprehensive primary health services, including their ability to diagnose and treat common illnesses and injuries, NPs are uniquely prepared to meet the needs of underserviced communities. Nurse practitioners can play an important role in managing sexual and reproductive health, family violence, lifestyle issues, and breast and cervical cancer screening, to name a few. In order to meet the local and cultural needs of communities, underserviced communities including ethnocultural groups, would be encouraged to identify, within their communities, RNs who have potential to become NPs, to encourage and support them to enter the NP educational program, and to return to the community to provide services.

Within underserviced communities, NPs can be placed in nursing stations, public health units, small hospitals, health service organizations, community health centres, health clinics and collaborative, multidisciplinary group practices. They may also work with disenfranchised groups through shelters and food banks, and wherever health care is needed.

Governments must be aware of the possible ghettoization of nurse practitioners who may be seen as the provider useful mainly in remote areas of the country where physicians and other health care professionals are not willing to locate. This is one reason for the Ontario government's decision to place NPs in health care settings in all parts of the province, as NPs can be effective in providing primary health care services, community mental health services, emergency health services, long term care services, aboriginal health services, women and children's health services, as well as rehabilitation, substance abuse, diabetes, and cancer services. Pilot projects are needed to demonstrate the most effective use of NPs in providing primary health care. NPs have demonstrated their effectiveness in community health centres. Possible other settings may include NP-physician practice in small community settings, emergency room settings, NP practices linked to existing organizational units in communities with no physician or no access to care, and within aboriginal communities. With their focus on health promotion and disease/injury prevention, the NP's holistic, family-centred approach can play a vital role in improving the health of Canadians.

Fiscal Issues

If NPs are to be educated and employed, four key fiscal issues must be resolved:

Funding for the Education of Nurse Practitioners

Commitment to long-term funding for NP education is imperative. Funding is based on good health human resources planning where the need for NPs is demonstrated. Evaluation of the educational program is also essential to continued funding.

A Fair and Workable Way to Pay Nurse Practitioners

The remuneration of NPs poses the greatest challenge and potential barrier to placing NPs. Most governments would not support a fee-for-service remuneration mechanism. A salary on a scale of $60,000 to $80,000 per year has been recommended for NPs in Ontario.[61] Nurse practitioners are most likely to be hired by health agencies and institutions that have global budgets and pay workers on a salary basis. Governments need to critically examine and update policies concerning provider services, to support the integration of NPs in the health care system. Governments also need to develop, with regional planning bodies, a workable way to remunerate NPs in underserviced communities and to cover the cost of establishing and maintaining these practices.

Financial Disincentives in the Existing System

One great barrier to NPs working with family physicians is the existing fee-for-service system originally created to pay physicians and hospitals. The system does not encourage health promotion activities and does not support the use of other health professionals. As this system now operates, physicians, who delegate specific tasks and functions to NPs, charge the system for these tasks, and the public purse pays for both the physician's charges to the system and the NP's salary. Physicians who employ NPs must pay NPs' salaries out of their own billings to the health care system and this discourages the development of multidisciplinary primary health care teams and collegial practices. Furthermore, the existing system of remuneration limits the government in its ability to shift funds to pay NPs. If the health care system is to make more effective use of the skills of all health professionals, governments must establish both alternate payment systems and new corporate policies that will overcome the limitations of the current fee-for-service system and that will support and facilitate the integration of NPs and other health professionals into the health care team.

Financial Incentives for Nurse Practitioners

A number of nurses are already practising in remote or underserviced areas. However, if provinces want to attract a significant number of new NPs to practise in these communities, it may have to offer financial and other incentives now used to attract physicians to underserviced areas, such as extra pay, backup support, access to continuing education, and a certain number of paid trips out of the practice area.

Publicity and Public Relations

To provide effective care within their full scope of practice, NPs will need both public and professional support for their role. Consumers need to understand what NPs do and be willing to come to them for their care. In addition, NPs need colleagues in other professions, to work with them in an equal partnership, to refer clients to them, and to accept their referrals. Currently, the public and many professionals do not understand the full role of the registered nurse, let alone that of the nurse practitioner. To support NPs in their work, there must be an organized program of public relations and education. The target audiences for education should be those who hold the power and/or influence how nurse practitioners will practise and those who will use the services of the NP. To ensure consumers will come to nurse practitioners for health services, the public must understand the role of the NP and the benefits of going to her/him for care. To increase public awareness, both government and the profession may want to design strategies which address the nature of nursing and its role in society, the role of the NP in Canada's health care system, the benefits to consumers of having direct access to alternative primary health care providers, and examples of where NPs have made a real difference in the kind and quality of care received.

Education of Related Health Care Workers

To be equal partners on health care teams, nurse practitioners need the respect and support of other health care workers. Other providers often have the power to make it difficult for NPs to practise fully and effectively. Some physicians, particularly family physicians, have already expressed their concern about NPs. Many do not understand the nurses' scope of practice. They are reluctant to acknowledge the overlap between medicine and nursing or to see activities already carried out by existing NPs regulated by laws that would remove the need for physicians to delegate certain acts. Other allied health professionals may be more accepting, but are often misinformed about the role of the NP.

In educating our colleagues in other professions, it must be emphasized that independent clinical decision-making does not preclude collaboration. There is a great deal of confusion around the concept of independent decision-making, especially in the overlap between nursing and medicine and collaborative practice. Some health professionals believe that NPs working as independent decision-makers will therefore not be collaborating with other members of the health care team. (Fig 6)

Education of Elected Officials, the Press and the Electronic Media

Elected officials, the press, and the electronic media have the power to shape opinions and to influence the impression that the public and other health professionals have of NPs. The nursing community needs to develop a coordinated education/public relations campaign aimed at these opinion shapers.

Education of the Nursing Community

The best spokes people for nurse practitioners are nurse practitioners themselves. The nursing community needs to know about the contribution made by nurse practitioners, but more importantly, that any gains made by NPs benefit the entire profession. Nursing also needs to develop a strategy to continue to lobby government and ensure NPs have the legislative changes and the support for education, placement, and remuneration systems which they need to practise effectively.

Figure 6
Overlap Between Medicine and Nursing

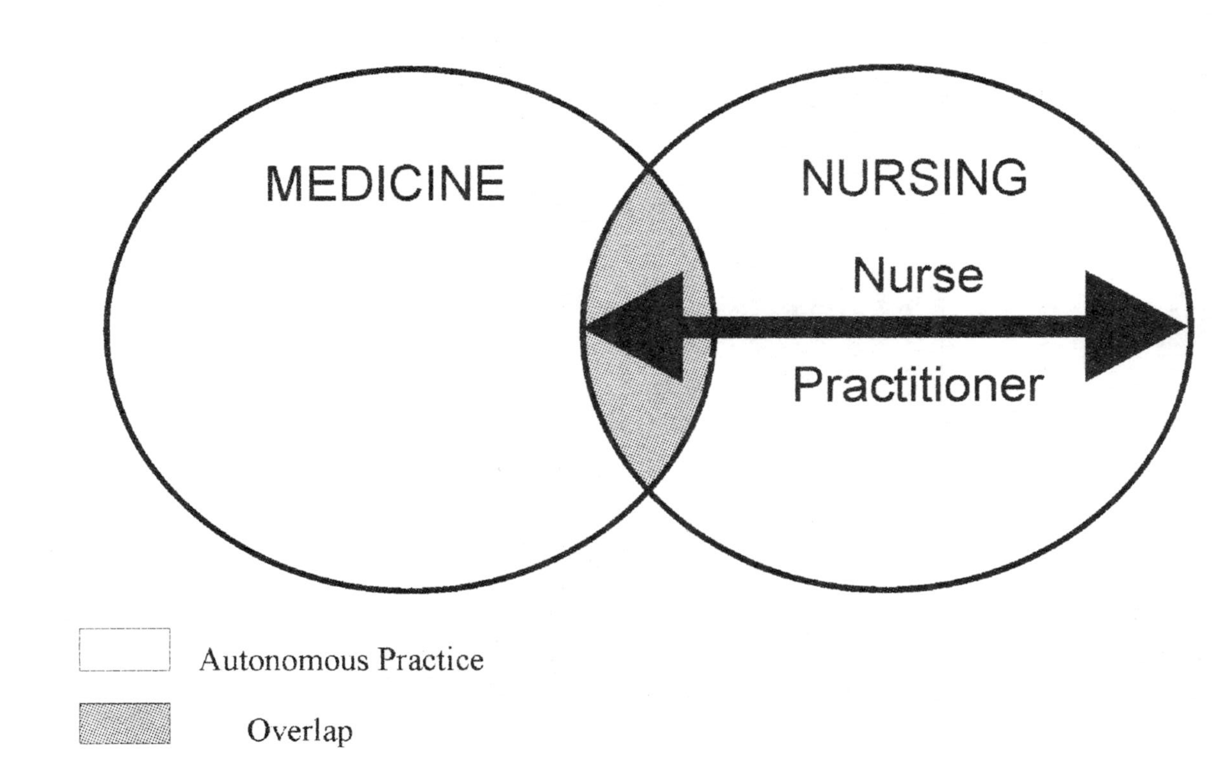

Evaluation

Although NPs are not new to Canadian health services, the NP will be under scrutiny as she/he is being reintroduced in our health care system. To ensure that the NP initiative is properly assessed, to determine whether it has achieved its objectives and to guide the education and employment of NPs in the future, governments will need to consider the evaluation of the following: clinical practice outcomes, including the impact on clinical outcomes and service utilization, and practice educational outcomes, including prior learning assessment (PLA) outcomes, education costs, and other important outcomes related to whether the NP program meets the needs of the learners and of the communities which they serve; placement outcomes, including mix and distribution of NPs, barriers to placement, impact on client satisfaction, on the health care system, and on other health professions; and fiscal considerations such as cost effectiveness.

It is crucial to measure the nursing contribution made by NPs rather than simply comparing the NP's performance to that of the physician. The evaluation must be rigorous in its design and methodology to withstand the scrutiny of the medical community and to be credible in order to provide direction for the further education and employment of NPs. A five-year evaluation of the NP initiative has been funded to examine the aforementioned structures, processes, and outcomes.

Conclusion

We are at the dawn of a new era in health care in Canada. Although the health care system will continue to be limited by scarce fiscal resources, the opportunities for new, different, and effective models of health care, and for new ways of delivering care, are emerging. Keeping Canadians healthy through health promotion and disease prevention has become a priority, and providing citizens with options regarding provider of care, such as the NP, is now a reality. The fact that nurses, including NPs, have been underutilized is beyond dispute. This is an opportunity to make the best use of nursing knowledge, and for nursing to emerge as a profession which is recognized for its impact on the health care system.

The nursing community must promote the diversity in the profession and, therefore, support the role of the NP. All of nursing will benefit from the successful reintegration of NPs into Canada's health care system.

Nursing must remain unified and focused on a changing health system which values the individual's, family's and community's participation in decisions about health care and health care delivery. Nursing must work at influencing healthy public policy which is caring in nature. Governments can no longer provide answers to the complex problems in our health care system in isolation. Nursing must be there to guide and assist governments in their decisions, especially in these uncertain times.

Acknowledgement

We wish to acknowledge the contributions made by Alba (Mitchell) DiCenso, Janet Pinelli and Chris Patterson for the section dealing with health care reform.

Chapter Eight

From a Community Perspective: Community Nurse Practitioners in Alberta

Karen Titanich

Introduction

In Alberta, the role of the community nurse practitioner emerged from the need to improve access to health services for specific underserviced communities in rural Alberta. In response to unforeseen reductions in already episodic and fragmented health services, five communities asked for assistance from Alberta Health to improve their health services. As a result, in 1992, Alberta Health established two project teams to consider alternative ways of improving access to a broader range of health services for these five communities located in two areas of northern Alberta. These small communities did not have hospitals, had difficulty attracting or retaining physician services, and had sporadic and limited access to other health services.

The purpose of the alternate health services delivery projects was to assist the five communities in planning for coordinated, integrated community-based health services. The project teams examined the broad issues related to the determinants of health and the root causes of disease and injury. In addition, they considered ways to improve access to needed health programs and services by developing community-based programs and services which could be coordinated with other services available at the district, regional, and provincial levels.

Community-based programs and services would address the community's particular needs for health promotion, health protection, disease and injury prevention, support, treatment, and rehabilitation. Referral to health services located outside the community and access to emergency services, including stabilization, and transport to other health services when needed, were also considered.[1]

The five interested communities, agencies responsible for health services delivery, and other stakeholders including local politicians, agreed to participate in community-based planning projects to assess their needs, and develop proposals to address them. There was agreement that the key service provider would be a registered nurse. A registered nurse could be capable of providing or co-ordinating a full range of primary health care services to meet community needs. This was an important consideration, since the registered nurse might be the only health professional in a particular community.

Principles and Concepts

The community-focused projects built upon the principles of primary health care and the inherent concepts of health promotion and community mobilization and development.[1] Key concepts that guided the planning process were:

Health
It is "the extent to which an individual or group is able, on the one hand, to realize aspirations and satisfy needs, and on the other hand, to change or cope with the environment. Health is therefore seen as a resource for everyday life, instead of as the objective of living."[2]

Population Health Needs
The focus will be on the health needs and priorities of the community.

Health Outcomes
Health programs and services will be evaluated for their contribution to the improved health of the population served.

Sensitivity to Aboriginal Health and Cultural Needs

Primary Health Care
The Alma Ata Declaration and its application, as described in World Health Organization documents, defined the concepts of primary health care which guided the project. Primary health care is "essential health services based on practical, scientifically sound, and socially acceptable methods and technology made universally accessible to individuals and families in the

community at a price they can afford to maintain at every stage of their development in the spirit of self-reliance and self-determination. It forms an integral part both of the country's health system, of which it is the central junction and main focus, and of the overall social and economic development of the community. It is the first level of contact of individuals, the family and community with the national health system, bringing health services as close as possible to where people live and work, and constitutes the first element of a continuing health process."[3]

There are six principles imbedded in the definition of primary health care:

- provision of essential health services;
- contact point for consumers with the health system;
- full participation of individuals and the community;
- accessible health services;
- intersectoral collaboration; and
- socially acceptable and affordable methods and technologies.

Health Communities: The Process

A planning process has been developed to use when working with communities which guided the steps in these projects.[4] (Table 5)

Development of community services involved adapting, integrating, and applying these concepts and principles, which had not been used before, to support the design of holistic community-based health service delivery. These concepts and innovative methods of assessing, planning, implementing, and evaluating programs and services to meet population health needs were also consistent with health system restructuring and the need to rebalance the health workforce. Duo to the organization of health services in Alberta at that time, this was the first time integrated, community-focused service delivery was planned in Alberta.[5]

Table 5

Overview of the Process

PHASE OF THE PROCESS	FOCUS OF ATTENTION	MAJOR TASKS DURING THIS PHASE
ENTRY PHASE	• The existing situation	• Learn about the environment within which the process will happen. • Introduce yourself into that environment.
NEEDS ASSESSMENT PHASE	• Health Needs	• Gather facts and opinions about community health needs. • Learn what skills and resources already exist.
	• Public Acceptance	• Have key individuals and the public accept that health needs are significant. • Gain commitment to action.
PLANNING PHASE	• How to respond to health needs	• Explore and choose methods of responding to the health needs. • Acquire necessary resources.
DOING PHASE	• Community action	• Implement plans.
RENEWAL PHASE	• Evaluation /Rejuvenation	• Evaluate what worked, what didn't. • Determine what has been learned. • Foster self-renewal of those involved. • Re-examine the existing situation.

Health System Restructuring in Alberta

The need for health system restructuring has been recognized in Alberta for at least a decade. The first step was the creation of the Premier's Commission for Future Health Care for Albertans in 1986. The Commission report, released in 1990, Rainbow Report: Our Vision for Health,[6] identified five principles to guide health system reform.

People →	We believe in people being the focus of the health system.
Choice →	We believe in free and voluntary individual choice, personal responsibility, and duty to others.
Change→	We believe in the inevitability and desirability of change, and in our ability to manage change to accomplish our purposes.
Decisions→	We believe in health decisions which are most effective and least intrusive.
Opportunity→	We believe in making the opportunity available to all Albertans to maximize their own health.

To achieve their vision of "healthy Albertans living in healthy Alberta," the commission proposed several directions for change:

- Government committing to the health of its people as a priority.

- Albertans taking more responsibility for becoming and remaining healthy.

- Governments returning the authority for decisions affecting the relevance of health services to people within the communities, familiar with local needs and priorities.

- Albertans having realistic expectations regarding living and dying.

The Government of Alberta's response to the Rainbow Report titled: Partners in Health[7] agreed that the health system would need to adapt to meet the changing health needs of Albertans in an affordable manner. Major changes for the future included:

- more prevention and less need for treatment;

- less institutionalization and more home and community care;

- more effective and co-operative use of health professionals and fewer boundaries among disciplines;

- more attention to outcomes and results;

- funding systems based on goals and accountability; and

- the importance of partnerships.

Another important Canadian policy document released in 1991, by Barer and Stoddart, was entitled Toward Integrated Medical Resource Policies for Canada.[8] This report highlighted our resistance to changing directions, even when such redirection is clearly called for. It pointed to the need to consider physician resource policy within the broader context of health and social policy. Eliminating exclusive fields of practice and increasing emphasis on alternative services or delivery models to improve population health were key recommendations.

In 1993, the Government of Alberta made a commitment to eliminate the provincial deficit over four years. This decision had implications for the health sector and added impetus to fundamentally restructure the health system. Given that over 70% of the health budget goes to salaries, benefits and payment of health industry workers, Albertans recommended that health human resources be managed more efficiently. Recognizing that health expenditures had to be reduced while maintaining and improving the health of Albertans, the government held a series of round tables for additional public consultation. As a result, Starting Points: Recommendations for Creating a More Accountable and Affordable Health System[9] was released in December 1993. The document charted a course for implementing a vision of Alberta's health system. Themes addressed in the document were putting the consumer first; creating health regions to enhance local decision-making; defining and communicating the roles of health system partners, including government, the regions, providers, and consumers to improve accountability; establishing guidelines to ensure compensation fair to both health professionals and taxpayers; and identifying a plan for restructuring the system.

Another pivotal document, Health Goals for Alberta: Progress Report,[10] was released in December 1993. The report presented a vision of health, nine health goals for Alberta, and the objectives and priorities to meet these goals. Four main challenges were identified:

- Maintaining the quality and accessibility of health care services in a time of rapid social and economic change.

- Maintaining and improving the good level of health the population enjoys, and responding to the needs of older Albertans as the population ages.

- Ensuring equitable access to opportunities to improve health for groups and communities not currently experiencing levels of health as good as most other Albertans.

- Ensuring a capacity to respond effectively to new health issues and needs that may emerge in the years ahead.

The first Alberta Health Three-Year Business Plan,[11] released in February 1994, outlined the steps which would be taken to make Alberta's health system responsive, contemporary, and affordable. Number seven, a key principle, stated that Alberta Health would encourage the use of appropriate services at the least cost by a range of qualified providers

In April 1994, boundaries were established for 17 health regions in Alberta. According to the *Regional Health Authorities Act*,[12] proclaimed in 1994, the health regions shall:

- promote and protect the health of the population in the health region and work towards the prevention of disease and injury;

- assess on an ongoing basis the health needs of the region;

- determine priorities in the provision of health services in the region and allocate resources accordingly;

- ensure that reasonable access to quality health services is provided in and through the region; and

- promote the provision of health services in a manner that is responsive to the needs of individuals and communities and supports the integration of services and facilities in the region.

The legislation also requires the Regional Health Authorities to establish community health councils. Regional Health Authorities receive public funds from the provincial government to carry out their responsibilities.

Community nurse practitioners, with their focus on the population health of communities, will be participating in health services planning, implementation, and evaluation based on the new business planning process for the restructured health system. The business planning process includes assessing community needs, determining goals and desired results, setting priorities and allocating resources (including the number and mix service providers), implementing programs and services and evaluating results. Community residents are expected to be a integral part of the process throughout.

Planning for the Introduction of Community Nurse Practitioners

While the communities were developing their proposals, the role of the community nurse practitioner was determined by an interdisciplinary working group which developed the

Guidelines for Registered Nurses in Advanced Nursing Practice Providing Primary Health Care Services in Underserviced Communities in Alberta.[13] The interdisciplinary working group included representatives from the Alberta Association of Registered Nurses, the College of Physicians and Surgeons of Alberta, the Alberta Pharmaceutical Association, the College of Family Physicians of Canada (Alberta Chapter), the Consumers' Association of Canada (Alberta), Medical Services Branch of Health Canada, practising registered nurses and Alberta Health. The document was developed to support alternate health services delivery projects in Rainbow Lake and the northern communities of Loon Lake, Peerless Lake, Red Earth Creek, and Trout Lake. The working group recognized that there were other communities in Alberta which could benefit from a similar community-based approach to health services.

The guidelines document was intended to clarify the role of registered nurses who would be providing primary health care services in underserviced communities and their relationship with other service providers. The working title 'community nurse practitioner' was chosen to reflect the larger, advanced community health nursing aspects of the role as well as the areas of assessment, diagnosis, treatment, drug therapy and referral which are shared with physicians, pharmacists, and other service providers. These community nurse practitioners would focus on the population health of their communities while providing entry-level diagnosis and treatment, referral and access to emergency services for individuals and their families when needed. These registered nurses would be able to carry out comprehensive health assessments; order and perform screening and diagnostic tests, diagnose and treat common disorders which affect children and adults; and access ground and air ambulances and other emergency services. They would be able to identify and manage common medical disorders affecting adults and children, common gynaecological and obstetrical disorders, common psychosocial/mental health problems, common occupational injuries, as well as emergency situations. These registered nurses would be autonomous practitioners who would recognize their limitations and refer those people who have conditions requiring different expertise to appropriate practitioners.

Specific procedures and activities related to managing common disorders affecting the health of adults and children would be subject to agency policy, staff competency, availability of support systems, client requirements, and the professional judgment of the community nurse practitioner. It was considered essential that diagnostic groups and cases beyond the capacity of the particular practice setting would be designated for referral to appropriate service providers and agencies.

With regard to referrals, community nurse practitioners would consult and refer as needed to the other members of the primary health care team, (e.g., dietitians, mental health therapists, physical therapists, family physicians, and pharmacists). The needs of clients might also require referrals to specialized services. Whenever possible, community nurse practitioners would make these referrals to other service providers and other service levels in consultation with family physicians and other health service providers.

Community nurse practitioners would use their professional judgment in the management of emergency situations. They would access air and ground ambulance services directly when necessary. The employing agency would develop and maintain an ongoing network and structure which facilitates referrals.

The employer would have the responsibility to establish the scope of services provided by the agency and the functions of employees. Considering the following factors would be helpful when carrying out this responsibility:

1) community needs,
2) geography,
3) the availability of support system,
4) professional legislation and AARN Standards of Practice and Position Statement and services legislation,
5) competency of the community nurse practitioner,
6) interdisciplinary co-operation and coordination of activities,
g) full participation of clients, families and community, and
8) public safety.

Employers would also have the responsibility to establish and maintain the infrastructure (policies, procedures, support personnel, equipment, referral mechanisms, and information and communication systems) needed for the delivery of primary health care services.

Enabling Factors for Implementation of the Role

Although registered nurses have been carrying out aspects of this new role for many years, barriers have prevented competent and qualified registered nurses from practising to the full extent of their abilities. Registered nurses have been granted delegated authority to provide the treatment and emergency services usually provided by physicians and pharmacists. Most of the nurses working in this role within Alberta are employed by Medical Services Branch, Health Canada. Within the provincial health system, few registered nurses provide these services. Over time, the role has almost disappeared as sectors responsible for health services fragmented delivery. Public health services became distinct, from the medical treatment and emergency services provided by physicians, pharmacists, ambulance services, and hospitals. This fragmentation was not conducive to integrated and coordinated health services planning and delivery.

The recommendations to restructure the health system, along with the need to improve access to health services for specific underserviced communities in Alberta, provided an opportunity to re-examine the role. Enabling community nurse practitioners to practise autonomously will require changes in both health professional and health services legislation and regulations, as well as the development of an accessible education program to prepare community nurse practitioners.

A. Legislative Changes

The Peace River Health Unit and the Northwestern Health Services Region, involved in the community projects, lobbied the provincial government for legislative authority to implement the envisioned role of the community nurse practitioner. It was known that section 21(l) of the *Public Health Act* [14] afforded authority for community health nurses to provide the preventive, treatment, and emergency services permitted in the regulation. However, the regulations were never developed, and this section did not come into use.

Since the section existed and afforded the authority needed, the decision was made to amend the *Public Health Act.*[14] The amendment to the *Public Health Act* [14] reflected the change in title of these nurses and the types of health services that would be provided. The Alberta Association of Registered Nurses coined the term 'registered nurse providing extended health services,' since these are additional services to those described in the scope of practice and beginning competencies for registered nurses. The term also became the title of the regulation required pursuant to section 21 of the *Public Health Act.*[14]

The February 1995 Speech from the Throne included the government's intention to amend the *Public Health Act*[14] to enable the role of the community nurse practitioners. Bill 5 was tabled in the Legislative Assembly on April 3, 1995, by Ms. Pearl Calahasen, Member of the Legislative Assembly for Lesser Slave Lake, where the northern communities are located. This amendment was not proclaimed and was subsequently replaced by the *Public Health Amendment Act* 1996, which also provided the needed authority for the regulation.

Alberta Health developed the required *Registered Nurse Providing Extended Health Services Regulation*[15] in collaboration with stakeholders, including the Alberta Association of Registered Nurses (AARN), the Alberta Pharmaceutical Association, and the College of Physicians and Surgeons of Alberta. Specifically, the regulation identified the extended health services which these registered nurses may provide, such as diagnosis and treatment of common disorders affecting the health of adults and children, referral, and emergency services. The regulation references the guidelines document to provide the context for the regulation.

The Registered Nurse Providing Extended Health Services Regulation received cabinet approval on September 24, 1996. Section 9 of the *Public Health Amendment Act* and the regulation came into force on October 1, 1996.

This regulation provides Regional Health Authorities with an option when considering the delivery of health services to underserviced communities in their regions. Community nurse practitioners will be either employed or contracted by Regional Health Authorities. The Minister of Health has been granted the authority to approve the communities where Regional Health Authorities may deploy community nurse practitioners.

In addition, these nurses cannot be hired unless the Alberta Association of Registered Nurses (AARN) is satisfied as to the registered nurse's competence to provide extended health services. In order to meet this requirement, the AARN has developed Competencies for Registered Nurses Providing Extended Health Services.[16] The AARN will be establishing the processes and mechanisms needed to assess the competency of these nurses and to recognize them over the coming months.

Other legislative changes are needed to enable community nurse practitioners to perform and order screening and diagnostic tests and to receive and analyse the results, to manage persons with communicable diseases and to notify as required, and to access ground and air ambulances. Specifically, changes have been made to the Medical Profession Bylaws of the College of Physicians and Surgeons of Alberta to authorize physicians to accept orders for tests from and send results to community nurse practitioners. Other changes identified include the Communicable Disease Control Regulations of the *Public Health Act*[14] to ensure these nurses would be required to make notifications and have the authority to manage communicable diseases. The Licensing Regulation pursuant to the *Ambulance Services Act*[17] has been identified for change to enable community nurse practitioners to direct the destination of a patient being transported by ambulance. The new *Pharmaceutical Profession Act*[18] does not need to be changed, since it is enabling and allows for practitioners authorized in legislation to prescribe drugs.

It is not known whether or not these particular changes will go forward as described, since a major review of all health services legislation and regulations has recently been initiated. The review is intended to streamline legislation and eliminate unnecessary regulations. The outcome is expected to be enabling legislation and regulation.

B. Education

Until recently, there was not an educational program in Alberta which could prepare registered nurses for the role of community nurse practitioner. However, Athabasca University's Centre for Nursing and Health Studies received funding through the Health Workforce Education Project to design a post-baccalaureate Advanced Graduate Diploma in Community Nursing Practice program (AGD:CNP).[19]

Before the detailed outlines for the course work were developed, site visits were made to Ontario and Nova Scotia in September 1995 to learn more about educational programs for nurse practitioners offered in these jurisdictions. A new program in Ontario was being developed through a consortium of university nursing programs. The first students had entered the program that month. Two programs funded by Medical Services Branch, Health Canada were also visited: the Northern Community Nursing Program at McMaster University in Hamilton, Ontario, and the well known Outpost and Community Health Nursing Program at Dalhousie University in Halifax, Nova Scotia. As a result, Athabasca University program graduates will have similar knowledge, skills and abilities as the graduates of the other programs. These similarities will promote graduate mobility across the country.

The Athabasca University program will address the academic and clinical preparation of nurses whose role will focus on advanced community health nursing practice and the provision of extended health services in primary care. Emphasis will be placed on ensuring the acquisition of skills and knowledge required for assessment, diagnosis, intervention, therapeutics and management of individuals, families and communities within a primary health care framework which emphasizes community development and health promotion. The entire program of studies will be offered through a combination of distance delivery methods to both full-time and part-time students. All the course work, with the exception of the final integrative practicum, can be challenged.

A multidisciplinary advisory committee has been established to assist Athabasca University in the development of the program. The advisory committee includes the Alberta Association of Registered Nurses, the College of Physicians and Surgeons of Alberta, the Alberta Pharmaceutical Association, health authorities, Alberta Health, educators, and nurses educated as nurse practitioners. The first students entered the program in 1997.

C. Community and Consumer Support

While legislative and education changes are needed to implement the role, the crucial enabling factors were the expressed needs by the communities for improved access to health services and their willingness to participate in a partnership to develop coordinated, integrated community based health services. Ms. Pearl Calahasen, Member of the Legislative Assembly for Lesser Slave Lake, also championed the cause of the northern communities. In August 1993, the Honourable Shirley McClellan, Minister of Health, visited Peerless Lake and expressed her support for the communities' efforts to improve their health services.

The communities have been partners every step of the way. The examples which follow illustrate how they have participated and driven the process. Their lobbying helped to garner political support for a new approach to meeting their health needs. They examined their health needs and helped to develop the community-based proposals to meet them. The Rainbow Lake Community Health Liaison Committee, which represented the community residents during the proposal development process, has been transformed into the Community Health Council for Rainbow Lake, as required under the *Regional Health Authorities Act.*[12] The northern communities each participated in selecting the registered nurse who would live and work in their community. The success of these projects, including the implementation of the community nurse practitioner role, depends upon the continuing input, feedback, commitment and support that the citizens of these communities have demonstrated. The importance of their continued participation cannot be overemphasized.

D. Reimbursement

Reimbursement of community nurse practitioners within the provincial health system will vary depending upon the Regional Health Authority and the specific circumstances. Those registered nurses who are employees and members of a bargaining unit will receive a salary and benefits according to the labour-management agreement. Those contracted to provide services will negotiate their reimbursement as will those in management positions. There is no provision for community nurse practitioners in Alberta to be paid through fee-for-service. Alternative payment arrangements to fee-for-service are being considered as part of health system restructuring. In addition, the Alberta Association of Registered Nurses considers salary and contractual arrangements to be reasonable reimbursement mechanisms for their members.

Lessons Learned

Strengths of this initiative continue to be its purpose, and the process used to develop the various aspects of the initiative. Improving access to health services for underserviced communities in Alberta is a purpose worthy of our efforts which everyone can understand. The clear purpose serves to keep the initiative on track. The participating communities have taken on the challenge of working in partnership and have made significant contributions to the development of health services in their communities. As well, working collaboratively has meant that varying perspectives can be considered as the initiative unfolds. With regard to the role of the community nurse practitioner, having representatives of the College of Physicians and Surgeons of Alberta, the Alberta Pharmaceutical Association and the Alberta Association of Registered Nurses participate from the beginning has proved invaluable. These regulatory bodies have shared information about the initiative with their memberships and helped to correct misunderstandings which have occurred from time to time.

Next Steps

Where to from here is an interesting question. In the short term, the communities with approved projects will be looking forward to implementing the role of the community nurse practitioner once the legislative authorities are in place. In all cases, interested nurses will be assessed by the Alberta Association of Registered Nurses for their beginning competence in providing extended health services. Over the next few months, the AARN will be completing development of the processes needed for the assessment of competency and recognition of these nurses. For nurses interested in pursuing the role, the educational program at Athabasca University is up and running in 1997. Since it is offered through distance delivery, nurses who already live and work in underserviced communities in Alberta will be able to access the program. As well, Regional Health Authorities concerned about improving health services delivery in underserviced communities have another option available to them.

In the longer term, it is more difficult to predict what will happen. The Alberta government is committed to making the best use of the members of the health workforce. In November 1995, the Health Workforce Rebalancing Committee presented its findings and recommendations from their review of the regulation of health professions and occupations in Alberta to Ministers of Labour and Health. As stated in their final report, the principles and recommendations will provide the framework for creating a regulatory system to better enable Albertans to exercise freedom of choice of health providers within a range of safe options. By creating a uniform system of professional self-governance for all regulated health professions, the perceived hierarchy between professions will be lessened, and the transparency of the regulatory process and the accountability of regulatory bodies will be enhanced. *Principles and Recommendations for the Regulation of Health Professionals in Alberta: Final Report of the Health Workforce Rebalancing Committee*[20] has obvious implications for the potential deployment of community nure practitioners beyond underserviced communities in Alberta. The pivotal recommendation is the removal of exclusive scopes of practice, making deployment of community nurse practitioners easier for Regional Health Authorities. As rebalancing the health work force to support health system restructuring progresses, it will be known whether or not the potential will be realized.

Chapter Nine

Legal Implications of Practice: An Overview

Leah Parisi

Nurses are governed by laws, regulations and policies in both their personal and professional lives. This chapter will assist the nurse to acquire a greater understanding of the legal system, the aspects of law which affect nursing practice, and the developing nature of laws and policies which guide advanced nursing practice. Since nursing practice is regulated by the province in Canada (the state in the United States), laws may vary somewhat according to location. This chapter will deal with general principles of legal thought, giving examples from specific jurisdictions for illustration. It is incumbent on individuals to become familiar with the specific laws, regulations and policies applicable in their area of practice, whether they arise from statutes, the court system, or the employing agency.

The Legal System

Laws, which grow from societal customs and values, have developed in two forms: statutes, which are enacted by Parliament, provincial legislatures or municipal councils, and common law (case law), which is determined by judges and is based on precedent or principles determined in prior judicial cases.

Since statutes are enacted by publicly elected bodies, they may be viewed as an expression of public interest. The *Regulated Health Professions Act* (Ontario), *Nursing Professions Act* (Alberta), *Nurses Act* (Prince Edward Island, Quebec and New Brunswick), the *Registered Nurses Act* (British Columbia, Manitoba, Newfoundland, Saskatchewan) and the *Registered Nurses Association Act* (Nova Scotia), are examples of such statutes.[1] The Ministers of Health have the responsibility of administering these Acts. Usually this responsibility is delegated to the professionals governing bodies (e.g. College of Nurses). The College is then responsible for implementation of the A ct through its regulatory activities.[2]

Common law is made by judges when deciding disputes brought before them. The facts of a current issue in dispute are compared to the facts of prior cases, and principles of law settled in prior cases are applied to current disputes. An example of relevant common law is the Ontario case of *Malette v. Schulman*, which confirmed that in Ontario a patient's "right to refuse treatment is an inherent component of the supremacy of the patient's right over his own body."

In *Malette*, health care providers noted that the plaintiff, who was a Jehovah's Witness, carried a card indicating that no blood was to be given. In the opinion of the physician, administration of blood was believed to be in the patient's best interest and blood was given. The Court found that the patient had the right to refuse the blood (treatment) even though refusal increased the risk.[3] The Court's decision was based on a finding of battery, wherein the "course of treatment exceeds the consent given by the patient."[4] In battery, there may be no wrongful intent, and in contrast, there may be a sincere interest in helping the patient.

Statutory (legislated) and common (judge made) law are found in both public and private spheres. Public law includes constitutional law, the Charter of Rights and Freedoms, criminal law, and public regulation. The latter includes the regulation of nursing practice.

Private law encompasses contract law (breach of a promise), property law (conflict regarding ownership), and tort law (breach of a legal duty).

Tort law is further divided into intentional and unintentional categories. Intentional torts include assault, battery, false imprisonment, trespass, intentional infliction of mental suffering, interference with chattels (personal property), invasion of privacy and defamation (communication "which tends to injure reputation; to diminish the esteem, respect, goodwill, or confidence in which the plaintiff is held, or to excite adverse, derogatory, or unpleasant feelings or opinions against him").[5] Negligence, which is an unintentional tort, is a common allegation in malpractice actions against health care practitioners. Negligence will be discussed in further detail subsequently.

Institutions or agencies which enforce laws, regulations, or policies relating to health care providers include the civil courts, criminal courts, coroners' courts, and professional disciplinary bodies (e.g. College of Nurses). It is possible for a health care practitioner to be involved in a proceeding with more than one of these bodies in regard to the same issue. For example, if a patient is injured as a result of nursing practice, an allegation of malpractice may be brought in a civil court. At the same time, the College of Nurses may bring a disciplinary action against the nurse. As well, if there are allegations of a criminal nature, a criminal action might be brought by the Crown attorney (prosecutor).

In criminal cases, wherein loss of freedom, fines, or both are at issue, the prosecutor must prove the allegations beyond a reasonable doubt. In civil actions, the sanctions are usually monetary, and the standard of proof is based on the balance of probabilities. In professional disciplinary actions, the College bears the case, and the sanctions may involve licensure limitation or revocation.

Professional Status in Canada

In all provinces, if an individual is entered on the nursing register, that person is entitled to use the title, 'Registered Nurse.' Anyone who has not been entered on the register is not authorized to use the title. The recently implemented *Regulated Health Professions Act of Ontario*[6] (*Nursing Act*), states, "No person other than a member shall use the title registered nurse, or registered practical nurse, a variation or abbreviation or equivalent in another language." Named exceptions include 'Christian Science nurse' and 'graduate nurse.'[7]

The College of Nurses of Ontario is proposing two classes of nursing registration-the generalist and extended classes. The extended class is meant to recognize and regulate extended nurses, such as nurse practitioners (NPs). The requirements for holding an Extended Class Certificate include education and/or experience additional to that required for generalist practitioners. Lack of agreement as to the appropriate title(s) for advanced practice nurses and definition of the specialty(ies) and scope(s) of practice, as well as the cost of regulating more than one class, are among the reasons that title protection for nurse practitioners has not yet been implemented in any of the provinces.

In some provinces (Alberta, New Brunswick, Nova Scotia, Prince Edward Island, Saskatchewan and Quebec), statutes provide not only title protection to nurses but also prohibit non-registered individuals from practising nursing by granting an exclusive right to registrants to practise, pursuant to a specified definition of nursing practice. This is a right similar to the exclusive right to practise granted to physicians and dentists.[8] In the remaining provinces, statutes do not yet grant registrants an exclusive right to practise nursing, although the statutes do grant title protection, requiring that it is necessary to be a registrant to use the title, 'Registered Nurse.'

Nurse practitioners are educated to carry out activities, such as diagnosis, prescription, and treatment, which have traditionally fallen within the practice of medicine. If these activities are undertaken independently and without statutory authority, a nurse may be accused of violating the exclusive right to practise medicine, which is a right granted to physicians by statute. In both the United States and Canada, there have been challenges which allege the illegal practice of medicine by nurses. For example, in *Ducharme v. Royal Victoria Hospital*, wherein the practice of anaesthesia by nurses was challenged, the court held that the practice of anaesthesia by a nurse was not negligence per se.[9] The cases of *Chalmers-Francis v. Nelson* (California) and *Frank v. South* (Kentucky) both addressed the practice of anaesthesia by nurses and held that such practice was within the practice of nursing.[10,11] In contrast, nurses in extended roles have also been found to have acted outside of the practice of nursing. In *Argonaut Insurance Co. v. Continental Insurance Co.* (New York), a nurse was found to have acted beyond the scope of her duties, crossing the line "between nursing and medicine."[12] In *Hernicz v. State of Florida*, a nurse practitioner was found to have acted outside of the practice of nursing when ordering therapy and prescribing a medication without supervision by a physician.[13]

Today, most provinces have a statutory definition of nursing practice. If the activity of the nurse falls outside of that definition, and within the exclusive right of practice of another profession, a challenge may prevail. Therefore, it is imperative that both generalist and extended role nurses become familiar with the statutes and regulations which affect their profession and make sure that they practise within them. By doing so, they may avoid a legal challenge based on practice beyond the scope of nursing or, alternatively, be in the best position to prevail if such a challenge is presented.

Ontario Regulated Health Professions Act

In Ontario, under the Regulated Health Professions Act,[13] controlled acts were set forth, three of which can be performed by all registered nurses.[14] These acts include:

1. Performing a prescribed procedure below the dermis or a mucous membrane.
2. Administering a substance by injection or inhalation.
3. Putting an instrument, hand or finger,

    - Beyond the external ear canal,
    - Beyond the point in the nasal passages where they normally narrow,
    - Beyond the larynx,
    - Beyond the opening of the urethra,
    - Beyond the labia majora,
    - Beyond the anal verge, or
    - Into an artificial opening into the body. [15]

The statute requires that the registrant not undertake any of these activities unless ordered by a person authorized by the *Chiropody Act* (1991), *Dentistry Act* (1991), *Medicine Act* (1991), *Midwifery Act* (1991), or the activity is permitted by and performed in accordance with regulation.[16] Regulations which further define the Act may thus permit nurses to initiate specifically designated activities without an order.

In 1994, the Minister of Health of Ontario proposed that nurse practitioners (those holding an Extended Class registration) should be able to initiate the above acts, and further, should be permitted to carry out three additional acts:

1. Communicating a diagnosis or a disease or disorder as the cause of a person's symptoms.

2. Ordering the application of a form of energy as prescribed by regulation.

3. Prescribing a drug designated in regulations.[17]

The Minister attempted to avoid the lengthy process of legislative change by exercising a right pursuant to the *Regulated Health Professions Act* to exempt nurse practitioners from the limitations of the *Nursing Act*.[18] This would have permitted nurse practitioners to legally extend their practice to initiate certain acts without an order or without initiation pursuant to a medically delegated act. The Ontario Health Professions Regulatory Advisory Council reviewed the reasons both for and against this exemption, which was proposed to take place without legislative change, and found that "an exemption route serve(d) neither the public interest nor the best interests of any of those involved."[19] While determining that legislative change was necessary to permit extension of nursing practice, the Council recognized the 'extreme importance' of the issue of defining a scope of practice for nurse practitioners. Because of the importance of the issue, the Council stated that the legislative process is the process which is "commonly acknowledged to be the optimum route to usher in the type of changes currently under discussion."[19] In February 1998, the *Expanded Nursing Services for Patients Act* S.O. became law. This Act amends the Nursing Act by providing legal authority for nurses holding a certificate of registration to perform certain acts, in accordance with regulations, additional to those permitted under the general registration. In Alberta, legislation enabling extended practice for those registered nurses holding an extended certificate of registration came into effect in October 1996. Thus, nurses holding an extended certificate of registration must comply with the laws and standards set forth for all nurses, as amended by the pertinent provincial acts and all regulations under those acts.

Nurses practising in extended roles who do not hold the extended certificate of registration must comply with the laws and standards set forth for all nurses, regardless of additional educational and/or experience.

Change to a provincial nurse practice act must result from consideration of, and vote for, an amendment to the existing nursing act by elected members of the provincial parliament. This results in differences in the acts between provinces. Similarly, in the United States the statutes which dictate the scope of nursing and extended role nursing practice may vary considerably between states. As of 1994, "24 states require(d) physician supervision or collaboration for NPs to practice" and seven states were planning to introduce legislation which "would discontinue this requirement."[20] The most liberal states in terms of independent practice of extended role nurses are New Mexico and Alaska, which have defined advanced practice nursing in their nurse practice acts. In these states, advanced practice nurses are regulated by the state boards of nursing.[20]

Delegation

Until such time as the provinces define advanced nursing practice in statute, nurses carrying out extended roles must practise through the use of medical orders (a specific order for an individual patient) or directives. In Ontario, a medical directive has been defined as "a prescription for a procedure, treatment or intervention that may be performed for a range of clients who meet certain conditions. The medical directive identifies a specific treatment or range of treatments, the specific conditions that must be met, and any specific circumstances that must exist before the directive can be implemented."[21] The nurse who carries out a medical directive must possess the knowledge and judgment to understand when to implement the treatment, the possibility of risks involved, the possible outcomes, and have the skill both to implement the treatment and to manage the outcomes. If, in the nurse's judgement, assistance may be needed in management, the appropriate resources must be available to provide that assistance when the treatment is undertaken. The physician maintains responsibility for delegation of the act; however, the nurse may be accountable for his or her own actions in initiating the directive and in managing the outcome.[21]

In the usual circumstance, the use of medical directives should be approved by the senior administration and board of a facility/agency following discussion related to the types of procedures which may be initiated through a medical directive, as opposed to those which need orders specific to the individual. Additionally, policies should address the qualifications required of those authorized to initiate care through the use of medical directives.

An individual facility/agency may determine whether or not it will permit use of medical directives. If directives are used, a written document should define the specific procedure ordered, the conditions which must be met prior to implementation of the procedure, and the contraindications to the procedure. The written document should also include the signatures of both the authorizing physician and the approving administrator along with the dates of review.[21]

"The greatest legislative barrier currently facing NPs (nurse practitioners) is their lack of autonomy to practice."[22] Until such time as statutory changes are made which permit nurse practitioners to practise to the full extent of their education and capability, it must be remembered that current "laws are mandates, not suggestions," which require a 'must' and 'shall' intent.[23] Nurses must become familiar with their provincial nurse practice act, and the regulations which further define the act; they must confine their practice to the scope of the act and defining regulations regardless of whether personal education and experience have prepared them for a greater role. Additionally, nurses should be familiar with the policies of their employing agency or institution. Policies may differ from institution to institution and between specific settings within an institution. Such policies may legitimately limit practice within a specific organization even though such practice may be within the legal scope of the practice act. It is important to remain within the scope of practice permitted within a particular setting even if the individual is permitted to carry out a more extensive practice in a different employment situation. Rather than practising outside of the law or policy, the nurse should take a leadership role in proposing statutory and institutional policy change to permit practice at the maximum capability.

Negligence

All health care practitioners are concerned about avoiding allegations of malpractice. Although it is not always possible to avoid such allegations or claims, it is helpful to understand why a claimant or defendant may prevail in a malpractice action, so that if a claim is filed, the practitioner is in the best possible position to demonstrate that the care given was within the standard of practice.

In health care malpractice litigation, negligence is the predominant theory of liability. Negligence may be defined as "the omission to do something which a reasonable man, guided by those ordinary considerations which ordinarily regulate human affairs, would do, or the doing of something which a reasonable and prudent man would not do."[24] In this case, the reasonable man is seen as the reasonable nurse, or the reasonable extended role nurse.

In order to succeed in a negligence claim, the plaintiff (claimant) must prove, on the balance of probabilities, that:

1. A duty of care existed.
2. The nurse breached the duty of care.
3. Injury or damage occurred.
4. The specific breach was the cause of the damage.

Duty of Care

A duty of care arises when the event which occurs is reasonably foreseeable. In *Dowey v. Rothwell*, the court found that because the nurse was advised by the patient that she was about to have a seizure, yet the nurse failed to secure the side rails of the bed, the injury resulting from the patient's fall during the seizure was reasonably foreseeable. The nurse was found negligent in that she had a duty to the patient to raise the side rails.[25]

Breach of Duty
Breach of duty is established by showing that the nurse did not provide the usual care which should be provided by the reasonable nurse in similar circumstances. To do this, the plaintiff may show that the nurse did not comply with the policies, procedures, or usual practice of the employing agency or institution, or the usual standard of practice as demonstrated through the use of written professional standards, guidelines, regulations, and expert testimony. Nurses who have had like experiences may be called as experts by either the plaintiff or the defendant to testify as to their opinions regarding the nursing standard of practice in the circumstance at issue. Although to date, in Canada, the standard of care to which a nurse practitioner may be held has not been addressed by the courts, the experiences of courts in the United States, when dealing with issues of advanced practice nursing, may give guidance.

In *Planned Parenthood of Northwest Indiana, Inc. v. Vines,*[26] the court found that a nurse practitioner was a specialist, and therefore, was held to the standard of care of those practitioners with superior skill (skill exceeding that of a generalist nurse). A California court determined on different facts that a nurse's conduct was not measured by the standard of practice of a physician, but by other nurses in the same or similar circumstances.[27] Interpretation of these and similar case findings can be simplified to indicate that when a nurse practitioner is practising in the position and capacity of an advanced practice nurse, he or she would most likely be held responsible for the standard of care provided by the reasonable nurse practitioner in similar circumstances, as opposed to the standard of reasonable generalist nurse. If the practice of the reasonable nurse practitioner regarding the issue should be identical to that expected of a physician, the standard for both the nurse and the physician, as related to the specific issue, would most likely be the same. Likewise, if the standard of practice expected for the particular issue is that of the generalist nurse, as in a situation where the nurse is working in a position as a generalist and not in an extended role, the nurse practitioner may be held to the standard of the generalist nurse, and not to the higher standard. For example, Certified Registered Nurse Anaesthetists (CRNA) from the United States are educated and experienced in intubation. If a CRNA is currently working as a generalist nurse in a Canadian intensive care unit, and both the nursing practice act and the hospital policies and procedures do not recognize that nurses can perform endotracheal intubation, the nurse would most likely not be expected to intubate. As yet, however, the level of judgement required of the advanced practice nurse, practising in a non-advanced nursing situation, has not been settled by Canadian courts. Most likely the usual standard of practice of nurses in a similar generalist intensive care situation in Canada would be used by the court in arriving at a decision. In fact, if the nurse carries out a treatment or procedure which is outside of the scope of practice or job description for which the nurse was hired, she or he may be held responsible for any injury resulting from her/his own actions, if negligence is found. Additionally, the nurse may be subject to a claim of practising outside of the scope of nursing practice and, alternatively, practising medicine without a license. Therefore, it is in the best interest of nurses to be aware not only of the defined provincial scope of practice for which they are held responsible, but also to be aware of the policies of the employing agency/institution, the job descriptions under which they are employed and the standard of practice of nurses in similar circumstances.

In a study of nurse practitioners in the United States, all of whom stated that they had experienced malpractice claims filed against them, 50% of the claims related to failure to properly diagnose, and 42% related to negligent treatment.[28] Because nurse practitioners may be involved in decisions related to diagnosis or ruling out certain conditions, it is important to be aware of the need to refer to a physician when medical judgement is required. Although it has been recognized that nurses are responsible for independent actions, "the nurse still retains the obligation to make a referral when the situation calls for it, and the failure to do so (may) constitute(s) malpractice."[29]

Causation

There may be a situation in which a duty of care exists, that duty is breached by the nurse and damages are present, yet the breach of duty by the nurse did not cause the damage. For example, in *MacDonald v. York County Hospital*, nurses failed to report significant changes in a patient's condition to the physician. The physician testified that even if the nurses had called, it was doubtful that he would have taken action at that time.[30] Therefore, even though the nurses breached their duty, to notify the physician, that breach was not found to be the cause of the injury incurred by the patient, since the physician said that he would not have taken any further action even if he had been notified in a timely manner. It remains the plaintiff's burden of proof to demonstrate each of the four elements of negligence (duty of care, breach of that duty, causation [injury resulting from the breach of duty] and damages) in order to prevail in a negligence action.

Nurses in situations of alleged negligence are accountable to the nursing board or College in regard to the breach of the standard of nursing practice. This may have subsequent impact on the nurse's registration even if the plaintiff in a civil action did not prevail.

Of particular interest to physicians working with advance practice nurses is the potential for the physician to incur liability for the actions of the nurse. If the nurse is not the employee of the physician, some courts have found that the physician is not liable for the nurse's negligence unless the nurse is acting under the physician's 'control.'[31] In other cases, physicians have been held responsible, or partially responsible for a nurse's error.[32]

When different, or what seem to be conflicting findings are noted by different courts, the precedent set in the particular jurisdiction in which the proceeding is taking place prevails. It is important to realize that the facts of a particular situation may be similar or different from the precedent-setting case, and the amount of similarity and difference will influence the finding in the case at issue.

Vicarious Liability

If an employee is acting within the scope of his or her employment, an employer may be held responsible to the plaintiff for the injury. This concept is based on the legal doctrine of *respondeat* superior. The rationale for this doctrine is that the employer has the means to control the work of the employee, the employer obtains the benefit of the employee's work and, most likely, has access to greater financial resources from which to compensate the injured party. This doctrine, however, does not preclude responsibility and liability on the part of the nurse. If the nurse acts outside of the job description or scope of employment, for example, acting in an extended role when the job description calls for the practice of a generalist, or if the nurse acts intentionally, and harm to the plaintiff results, the nurse, and not the employer may be held responsible. Additionally, even though the employer may be responsible to the plaintiff, there is no reason that the employer cannot seek a judgement against the nurse for damages incurred from the nurse's negligence.

If a nurse is acting independently, outside of the scope of employment, or is in practice as an independent contractor, the nurse is responsible for her/his own actions. The nurse practitioner, therefore, must pay particular attention to whether her/ his actions fall within the scope of employment and within the relevant job description. If not, the nurse should refrain from such activity until such time as the extended activity is approved.

Consent

The ethical principle of autonomy is the basis of the client's right to accept or refuse treatment. This principle has been increasingly emphasized in recent years and the prior concept of paternalism, or the belief that the provider knows best as to what should be done, has been replaced by the patient's right to refuse treatment after adequate information has been provided, regardless of the risk inherent in refusal, and regardless of whether it is, in the opinion of the provider, in the best interest of the patient to undergo treatment.[33]

The elements necessary in informed consent include the capacity of the patient (or substitute decision maker) to understand the treatment, disclosure of the nature of the treatment proposed, the material effects, risks, side effects and alternatives, and voluntary consent.

It is important that not only the physician determine the material nature of the risks involved, but that the patient and family also be involved in that determination. The likelihood of risk may not be as important to the patient as the nature of the possible risk. For example, the risk of paralysis may be considered sufficiently material to a patient to warrant declining treatment, even though the likelihood of occurrence is small.[34]

Consent must be given voluntarily, and after the treatment, alternatives and risks have been explained at a level appropriate to the patient's comprehension. If a patient consents, then later refuses, the subsequent decision prevails. If the patient has questions, these must be clarified before the procedure is undertaken, and consent should be given subsequent to the clarification.

The physician performing the procedure has long been recognized as the individual with knowledge sufficient to give information and answer the patient's questions. Today expanded role nurses and other health care providers may decide upon and provide treatment. It is therefore necessary for these providers to obtain consent for treatment which they propose. If such consent is not informed and voluntarily obtained, yet a procedure is carried out which leads to injury, the plaintiff may prevail in battery. Alternatively, if the manner in which the information was given and the consent obtained does not fall within the usual standard of practice, the plaintiff may prevail in negligence.

Case law has demanded for over a quarter of a century that a patient must consent to treatment and must be given information which the reasonable person in similar circumstances would require in order to make a decision regarding consent. However, the Parliament of Ontario emphasized and extended the common law by passing the *Consent to Treatment Act*, which was implemented in 1995.[35] This act codifies the voluntary nature of the consent required, the requirements of capacity and the explanation of the risks and alternatives. If a health care provider does not comply with the requirements of the statute prior to carrying out a procedure, the provider may be found liable in battery, or alternatively, negligence.

It is recommended that the nurse practitioner not only comply with all required elements of informed consent, but also make sure that the client is aware of her/his professional status as a nurse practitioner. Misrepresentation as to professional status of the care provider may invalidate the consent. Providing this information not only assures that the patient understands the qualifications of the provider, but it also increases public awareness that nurses practise in extended roles.

Documentation

Health care records are used to communicate information to other health care providers as to the care and treatment given, to provide a record of care given as a historical reference, and to provide a record of the activities of the providers during treatment. The record may be the most reliable documentation of care, and thus may provide evidence for legal proceedings. After review, it will assist the provider to recall events and treatment. It will also be persuasive in regard to the accuracy of testimony in court.

Care should be documented at the time that it is provided, or as close to that time as possible. Immediate documentation will prevent inference that the record is not accurate because events may have been forgotten or memory blurred in the period between occurrence and charting. Information charted must be factual, specific, and related to care.

It is important, in most instances, that the individual who carried out an action be the one to record it. The events should be recorded in a clear factual manner, concisely detailing what was observed. Sufficient information should be included to allow the nurse to know, years later, exactly what he or she observed, and what actions were implemented. Abbreviations should be used only if they are generally acceptable, and their meaning is unmistakeable. Any corrections should be initialled and made by drawing a line through the words, permitting the previous statement to remain legible. The new entry should be accompanied by the date and time of documentation, as well as the signature of the recorder.

Documentation should be limited to care given. Opinions and judgements regarding care should not be included, unless they are directly related to the care provided. Information given by the patient, family, or others should be clearly identified and the source of the information recorded.

Provincial statutes document the length of time which records must be retained. The nurse practitioner should become aware of this statutory mandate, particularly if the nurse is in independent practice. Length of time for record retention varies between the provinces, and it is the responsibility of the provider to comply with the laws of the province in which she or he is practising.

Health care records are confidential. Although they may be used to communicate information relevant to care provided, this information must only be available to others directly involved in providing care, and the information obtained must be relevant to the care given. As computerized charting becomes more common, appropriate security measures must be implemented to ensure confidentiality.

The record itself is the property of the institution or care provider.[36] With written patient authorization, a record may be copied at the patient's expense. A court may also order production of records, a professional governing body may use a record for purposes of investigating a complaint, or in limited circumstances, records may be used for teaching and research. It is important that in all issues regarding records, as well as in a conversation regarding a patient, confidentiality of information be considered.

Contracts

The law of contracts is applicable to the nurse practitioner, as it is to all nurses, both professionally and personally. Although most actions against health care providers and hospitals are framed in negligence, it is possible that an action may be brought in contract. This is particularly true if there was a guarantee as to the result of care. In *LaFleur v. Cornelis*, the plaintiff underwent cosmetic surgery and was dissatisfied with the result. After the surgery, the patient sued, alleging breach of contract in that the physician advised her that she would be happy with the result, that he had contracted to use his best skills and had not done so, and that she had paid for the services. The plaintiff prevailed.[37] Similarly, if a nurse practitioner guarantees a result of her/his care, and that guarantee is not fulfilled, an action in contract could result.

Whether a health care claim is brought in contract or negligence depends on the facts of the case. The Supreme Court of Canada in *Cahoon v. Franks*, ruled that "the factual situation" determines whether a cause of action is in contract or negligence. Thus, for each individual factual situation there is only one right to sue.[38] A plaintiff will not be held liable in both contract and negligence in relation to the same issue.

The nurse practitioner may encounter contract issues in relation to patient care, but it is more likely that such issues will be encountered in relation to employment. Although it is recommended that a nurse have an employment contract in writing, even without a written document a contract may exist. The contract may be based on service provided for payment after a mutual understanding regarding employment was reached. It is the duty of the employee to provide service within the professional standards and the job description of the employer.

A nurse may also enter a contract with another individual in regard to forming a business venture or partnership. Further, at times third parties may contract services for another. The nurse should be aware of the benefits, responsibilities, and implications of contract formation and assure that the terms are not only clearly understood and agreed upon by the parties, but fulfilled.

Summary

This chapter is not intended to provide legal advice for given factual situations, nor is it inclusive of all aspects of law related to the areas discussed. It is meant to increase nurses' familiarity with the legal system, and to highlight areas having legal implications for nurse practitioners. The laws may differ between provinces, and between Canada and the United States. The illustrations used provide information on how courts have held in the past in given situations. Although common law precedent is usually followed in the same jurisdiction, a result may differ in different jurisdictions. In a similar manner, the statutory requirements of different jurisdictions may not be the same. It should also be understood that, at the time of this writing, nurses have not yet practised in legally recognized extended roles in most of Canada. Therefore, much of the discussion relates to findings from cases involving nurses in general, or those practising in recognized extended roles in the United States. As advanced practice nursing is further defined in provincial nurse practice acts and common law, answers to many questions may become clearer.

The nurse is advised to consult the statutes and law of the province in which she or he practises and, if questions arise, consult a professional lawyer.

References

Chapter 1

1. Pearson, L. (1985). Perspectives 20 years later: From the pioneers of the NP movement. *Nurse Practitioner* 10 (1): 15-22.

2. Kitzman, H.J. (1983) The CNS and the nurse specialist. In *The clinical nurse specialist in theory and practice*, ed., Hamric, A.B., & Spross, J., 275-289. New York: Grune and Stratton.

3. Mitchell, A., Pinelli, J., Patterson, C., & Southwell, D. (1993). *Utilization of nurse practitioners in Ontario: A discussion paper requested by the Ontario Ministry of Health*. Quality of Nursing Worklife Research Unit. McMaster University/University of Toronto, Working Paper Series 93-4.

4. American Association of Colleges of Nursing. (1995). 1994-1995 *enrollment and graduations in baccalaureate and graduate programs in nursing*. Washington, D.C.: American Association of Colleges of Nursing.

5. Bullough, B. (1992). Alternatives models for specialty nursing practice. *Nursing and Health Care* 13 (5): 254-259.

6. Mezey, M. (1993). Preparation for advanced practice. In *Nurses, nurse practitioners: Evolution to advanced practice*, eds., Mezey, M.D., & McGivern, D.O., 31-58. New York: Springer Publishing Company.

7. Alberta Association of Registered Nurses. (1995). Nurses: *Key to healthy Albertans*. Edmonton, Alberta: AARN.

8. Pearson, L. J. (1995). Annual update of how each state stands on legislative issues affecting advanced nursing practice. Nurse Practitioner: *The American Journal of Primary Health Care* 20 (1): 1-27.

9. Ontario Ministry of Health. (1994). *Nurse practitioners in Ontario*: A plan for their education and employment. Toronto: Queen's Printer for Ontario.

10. American Academy of Nurse Practitioners. (1994). Washington, DC.

11. OECD. (1995). *Program OECD health data.* OECD, Paris.

12. Evan, R.E. (1995). *Canada, Europe, and Expenditures on health care.* Paper presented to the National Forum on Health, Ottawa, Canada.

13. Evans, R.G ., Barer, M. L ., & Hertzman, C. (1991). The 20 year experiment: Accounting for explaining and evaluating health care costs containment in Canada and the United States. *Annual Review of Public Health* 12: 481-518.

14. Barer, B.L., & Stoddart, G.L. (1992). Toward integrated medical resource policies for Canada: Background, process and perceived problems. *Canadian Medical Association Journal* 146 (3): 347-351.

15. Manga, P., & Campbell, T. (1994). *Health human resource substitution: A major area of reform towards a more cost-effective health care system.* Queen's University of Ottawa Economic Projects, Working Paper 94-01.

16. Denton, F.T., Gafni, A., Spencer, B.G., & Stoddart, G.L. (1983). Potential savings from the adoption of nurse practitioners technology in the Canadian health care system. *Socio-Economic Planning Sciences* 17: 199-209.

17. Spitzer, W.O., Sackett, D.L., Sibley, J.C., Roberts, R.S., Gent, M., Kergin, D.J., Hackett, B.C., & Olynich, A. (1974). The Burlington randomized trial of the nurse practitioner. *The New England Journal of Medicine* 290 (5): 251-256.

18. Spitzer, W.O., Roberts, R.S., & Delmore, T. (1976). Nurse practitioners in primary care. V. Development of the utilization and financial index to measure effects of their deployment. *Canadian Medical Association Journal* 114: 1099-1102.

19. Spitzer, W.O. (1984). The nurse practitioner revisited: A slow death of a good idea. *The New England Journal of Medicine* 310 (16): 1049-1051.

20. Rachlis, M., & Kushner, C. (1989). *Second opinion: What's wrong with Canada's health care system and how to fix it.* Toronto: Harper & Collins Publishers Ltd.

21. Wilbur, J., Zoeller, L.H., Talasele, M., & Sullivan, J.A. (1990). Career trends of master's prepared family nurse practitioners. *Journal of the American Academy of Nurse Practitioners* 2 (2): 69-78.

22. United States General Accounting Office. (1994). *Report to the Chairman Committee on Government Operations, House of Representatives: Primary care physicians: Managing supply in Canada, Germany, Sweden, and the United Kingdom.* GAO 94-111, Washington, D.C.

23. McGivern, D.O. (1993). The evolution to advanced nursing practice. In *Nurses, nurse practitioners: Evolution to advanced practice*, (pp.3-30); eds., Mezey, M.D.,& McGivern, D.O., 3-10. New York: Springer Publishing Company.

24. Safreit, B.J. (1992). Health care dollars and regulatory sense: The role of advanced practice nursing. *Yale Journal on Regulation* 9 (2): 417-488.

25. Coghlan, A. (1995). President's message: Collaboration key to nurse practitioner role implementation. *College Communiqué* 20 (1): 4.

26. Health Professions Regulatory Advisory Council (1996). *Advice to the Minister of Health: Nurse practitioner referral.* Toronto: Queen's Printer for Ontario.

27. Alberta Association of Registered Nurses. (1995).*Competencies for registered nurses providing extended health services in the province of Alberta.* Edmonton, AB: AARN.

28. Alberta Association of Registered Nurses. (1991). *Nursing practice standards and competencies for nurses beginning to practice in Alberta.* Edmonton, AB: AARN

29. Evans, R. (1994). Introduction. In *Why are some people healthy and others not?*, eds., Evans, R.G., Barer, M.L., & Marmour, T.R., 3-26. New York: Aldine de Gruyter.

30. *A new perspective on the health of Canadians: A working document.* M. Lalonde, Minister of National Health and Welfare. Ottawa, Department of National Health and Welfare, 1974.

31. Pederson, A., O'Neill, M., & Rootman, I. (1994). *Health promotion in Canada: Provincial, national & international perspectives.* Toronto: W.B. Saunders Co.

32. O'Neill, M., Rootman, I., & Pederson, A. (1994). Beyond Lalonde: Two decades of Canadian health promotion. In *Health promotion of Canada: Provincial, national & international perspectives.* (pp. 374-386); eds., Pederson, A., O'Neill, M., & Rootman, I. Toronto: W.B. Saunders Co.

33. Mitchell, A., Patterson, C., Pinelli, J., & Baumann, A. (1995). *Assessment of the need for nurse practitioners in Ontario.* Quality of Nursing Worklife Research Unit. McMaster University/University of Toronto, Working Paper Series 95-7.

34. Zimmer, P.A. (1995, July). *NP issues update: Credentialing, certification, NP education, and "blended roles" in a reformed health care system.* Paper presented at the National Primary Care Nurse Practitioner Symposium, Keystone, Colorado.

35. Pearson, L.J. (1990). 25 years later. 25 exceptional NPs look at the movement's evolution and consider future challenges for the role. *Nurse Practitioner* 15 (9): 9-25.

36. Edmunds, M.W. (1988). Promoting visibility for the nurse practitioner role. *Nurse Practitioner* 13 (3): 53-55.

37. Nurse Practitioners' Association of Ontario, (1995). Nurse Practitioners' Association of Ontario: Position statement regarding title protection of the nurse practitioner. *NPAO in Action* 5 (2): 4.

38. Hanson, C., & Martin, L.L. (1990). The nurse practitioner and clinical nurse specialist: Should the roles be merged? *Journal of the American Academy of Nurse Practitioners* 2 (1): 2-9.

39. Elder, R.G., & Bullough, B. (1990). Nurse practitioners and clinical nurse specialists: Are the roles merging? *Clinical Nurse Specialist* 4 (2): 78-84.

40. Fenton, M.V., & Brykcyski, K.A. (1993). Qualitative distinctions and similarities in the practice of clinical nurse specialists and nurse practitioners. *Journal of Professional Nursing* 9 (6): 313-326.

Chapter 2

1. Mantle, J. (1993). Standards-will they make a difference? *The Canadian CNS: The Newsletter of the Clinical Nurse Specialist Group* 3: 1-8.

2. Mass, H., & McKay, R. (1995). Nurse practitioners: Expanding the role of nursing. *Nursing BC (August/ September)*: 7-9.

3. Patterson, C., & Haddad, B. (1992). The advanced nurse practitioner: Common attributes. *Canadian Journal of Nursing Administration* 5 (4): 18-21.

4. Mitchell, A., Pinelli, J., Patterson, C., & Southwell, D. (1993). *Utilization of nurse practitioners in Ontario: A discussion paper requested by the Ontario Ministry of Health*. Quality of Nursing Worklife Research Unit. McMaster University/ University of Toronto, Working Paper Series 93-4.

5. Alcock, D. (1994). *The clinical nurse specialist, clinical nurse specialist / nurse practitioner and other titled nurse in Ontario*. Unpublished manuscript.

6. Hunsberger, M., Mitchell, A., Blatz, S., Paes, B., Pinelli, J., Southwell, D., French, S., & Soluk, R. (1992). Definition of an advanced nursing practice role in the NICU: The clinical nurse specialist/neonatal practitioner. *Clinical Nurse Specialist* 6 (2): 91-96.

7. Van Der Horst, M-L., & Patterson, C.A. (1993). General medicine expanded role nurse: Role description. *Canadian Journal of Nursing Administration* 6 (3): 22-25.

8. Haddad, B. (1992). The development of the expanded role nurse: Background and questions surrounding the project. *Canadian Journal of Nursing Administration* 444: 6-9.

9. O'Rourko, M. (1989). Generic professional behaviours: Implications for the clinical nurse specialist role. *Clinical Nurse Specialist* 3: 128-132.

10. Storr, G. (1988). The clinical nurse specialist: From the outside looking in. *Journal of Advanced Nursing* 13: 265-272.

11. Coghlan, A. (1995). President's message: Collaboration key to nurse practitioner role implementation. *College Communiqué* 20 (1): 4.

12. Nurse Practitioners' Association of Ontario. (1995). Nurse Practitioners' Association of Ontario: Statement on independent practice. *NPAO in Action* 5 (2): 7.

13. Ford, L. (1979). A nurse for all settings: The nurse practitioner. *Nursing Outlook* 27: 516-521.

Chapter 3

1. Lee, H. (1991). Definition of rural: A review of the literature. In *Rural nursing*, ed., Bushy, A. Newbury Park, CA: Sage Publications.

2. Bigbee, J. (1993). The uniqueness of rural nursing. *Nursing Clinics of North America* 28: 131-143.

3. Long, K.A., & Weinert, C. (1989). Rural nursing: Developing the theory base. *Scholarly Inquiry for Nursing Practice: An International Journal* 3: 113-127.

4. Lee, H.J. (1993). Rural elderly individuals: Strategies for delivery of nursing care. *Nursing Clinics of North America* 28: 219-229.

5. Whitney, F.W. (1990). Nurse practitioners: Mirrors of the past, windows of the future. In *The nursing profession turning point*, ed., Chaska, N.L. Toronto: C.V. Mosby Co.

6. Mundinger, M. (1994). Advanced-practice nursing-good medicine for physicians. *The New England Journal of Medicine* 330: 211-214.

7. Weinert, C., & Long, K.A. (1990). Rural families and health care: Refining the knowledge base. *Marriage and Family Review* 15 (1-2): 57-75.

8. Fuszard, B. (1991). Future trends in nursing practice and technology. *The Journal of Rural Health* 7: 402-411.

9. Sutherland, R., & Fulton, J. (1994). *Spending smarter and spending less*. Ottawa: The Health Group.

10. Hastings, K.E. (1995). Health care reform: We need it, but do we have the national will to shape our future? *Nurse Practitioner* 20 (1): 52-57.

11. Devis, D.J., & Droes, N.S. (1993). Community health nursing in rural and frontier counties. *Nursing Clinics of North America* 28: 159-169.

12. Lassiter, P.G. (1985). Education for rural health professionals. *The Journal of Rural Health* 1: 23.

13. Haddad, B. (1987). *Expanded role nurse project.* Unpublished manuscript, University Hospital, Department of Nursing Services, London.

14. Haddad, B. (1992). Report on the expanded role nurse project. *Canadian Journal of Nursing Administration* 5 (4): 10-17.

15. Benner, P. (1984). *From novice to expert: Excellence and power in clinical nursing practice.* Menlo Park, CA: Addison-Wesley.

16. Mitchell, P. (1995). *Advanced nursing practice*, Address to AANN, Portland, Oregon.

17. Patterson, C., & Haddad, B. (1992). The advanced nurse practitioner: Common attributes. *Canadian Journal of Nursing Administration* 5 (4): 18-21.

18. Hunsberger, M., Mitchell, A., Blatz, S., Paes, B., Pinelli, J., Southwell, D., French, S., & Soluk, R. (1992). Definition of an advanced nursing practice role in the NICU: The clinical nurse specialist/neonatal practitioner. *Clinical Nurse Specialist* 6 (2): 91-96.

19. Paes, B., Mitchell, A., Hunsberger, M., Blatz, S., Watts, J., Dent, P., Sinclair, J., & Southwell, D. (1989). Medical staffing in Ontario neonatal intensive care units. *Canadian Medical Association Journal* 140. 1321-1326.

20. Mitchell, A., Watts, J., Whyte, R., Blatz, S., Norman, G., Guyatt, G., Southwell, D., Hunsberger, M., & Paes, B.(1991). Evaluation of graduating neonatal nurse practitioners. *Pediatrics* 88: 789-794.

21. Mitchell, A., Watts, J., Whyte, R., Blatz, S., Norman, G., Southwell, D., Hunsberger, M., Paes, B., & Pinelli, J. (1995). Evaluation of an educational program to prepare neonatal nurse practitioners. *Journal of Nursing Education* 24: 286-289.

22. Mitchell, A., Guyatt, G., Marrin, M., Goeree, R., Willan, A., Southwell, D., Hewson, S., Paes, B., Rosenbaum, P., Hunsberger, M., & Baumann, A. (1996). A controlled trial of nurse practitioners in neonatal intensive care. *Pediatrics* 98: 1143-1148.

23. Mitchell, A., Pinelli, J., & Southwell, D. (1996). Introduction and evaluation of an advanced nursing practice role in neonatal intensive care. In *Outcomes of effective management practice*, ed., Kelly, K., 171-186. California: Sage Publications.

24. Pinelli, J., & Paes, B. (1995). Advanced practice nurses in neonatal intensive care. In *Recent advances in pediatrics*, ed., David, T.J., 97-107. London: Churchill Livingstone.

25. Barnett, S., & Sellers, P. (1979). Neonatal critical care nurse practitioner: A new role in neonatology. *American Journal of Maternal Child Nursing* 4: 279-286.

26. National Association of Neonatal Nurses Board of Directors. (1995). Position statement on graduate education for entry into neonatal nurse practitioner practice. *Neonatal Network* 14: 52.

27. Canadian Nurses Association. (1986). *Position statement: Clinical nurse specialist.* Ottawa, ON: Canadian Nurses Association.

28. CanSig Board of Directors. (1995). *CanSig position on NNP education.*

29. Puterbough, C., & Love, B. (1981). *Paediatric nursing specialists: The role in action.* Unpublished manuscript.

30. Wolf, G. (1990). Clinical nurse specialists: The second generation. *JONA* 20 (5): 7-8.

31. Spitzer, W.O. (1984). The nurse practitioner revisited: A slow death of a good idea. *The New England Journal of Medicine* 310 (16): 1049-1051.

32. Dworkin, C. (1973). Spotlight on the clinical nurse specialist. *Canadian Nurse* 9: 40-42.

33. American Nurses Society: Oncology Nursing Society. (1990). *Standards of advanced practice in oncology nursing.* Pittsburgh, PA: Oncology Nursing Society.

34. Simpson, B. (1994). The acute care nurse practitioner programme: A collaborative effort. *Registered Nurse* 6 (6): 14-27.

35. Whitley, M. (1992). Characteristics of the expert oncology nurse. *Oncology Nursing Forum* 19 (8): 1242-1246.

36. Powel, L., & Mayer, D. (1992). The future of advanced clinical practice in oncology nursing. *Oncology Nursing Forum* 19 (1): 28-31.

37. Booth, R. (1995). Leadership challenges for nurse practitioner faculty. *Nurse Practitioner* 20 (4): 52-58.

38. El-Sherif, C. (1995). Nurse practitioner-where do they belong within the organizational structure of the acute care setting? *Nurse Practitioner* 20 (1): 62-65.

39. Capan, P., Beard, M., & Mashburn, M. (1993). Nurse-managed clinics provide access and improved health care. *Nurse Practitioner* 18 (5): 50-55.

40. Miaskowski, C. (1990). The future of oncology nursing: A historical perspective. *Nursing Clinics of North America* 25 (2): 461-473.

41. Williams, C.A., & Valdivieso, G.C. (1994). Advance practice models: A comparison of clinical nurse specialist and nurse practitioner activities. *Clinical Nurse Specialist* 8 (6): 311-318.

42. Anthony, W.A., & Liberman, R.P. (1986). The practice of psychiatric rehabilitation: Historical, conceptual and research base. *Schizophrenia Bulletin* 12 (4): 542-559.

43. Krauss, J.B., & Slavinsky, A.T. (1982). *The chronically ill psychiatric patient and the community.* New York: Blackwell Scientific.

44. Bullough, B. (1992). Alternate methods for specialty nursing practice. *Nursing and Health Care* 13 (5): 254-259.

45. American Nurses Association Council on Psychiatric and Mental Health Nursing. (1994). *Statement on psychiatric mental health clinical nursing practice and standards of psychiatric mental health clinical nursing practice.* Washington, D.C.: American Nurses Publishing.

46. Premier's Council on Health, Wellness, and Social Justice. (1990). *Mental health in Ontario: Selected findings from the mental health supplement to the Ontario health survey.* Ontario Ministry of Health.

47. Schreiber, R.S. (1995). (Re)*Defining my self. Women's process of recovery from depression.* Doctoral Dissertation, State University of New York at Buffalo.

48. Holbert, S., & Schreiber, R. (in press). *The role of the nurse in mental health reform.*

49. Slavinsky, A.T. (1984). Psychiatric nursing in the Year 2000: From a nonsystem of care to a caring system. *Image: The Journal of Nursing Scholarship* 16 (1): 17-20.

50. Sullivan, J.A., Dachelet, C.Z., Sultz, H.A., Henry, M., & Carrol, H.D. (1978). Overcoming barriers to the employment and utilization of the nurse practitioner. *American Journal of Public Health* 68 (11): 1097-1103.

51. Harrell, J.S., & McCulloch, S.D. (1986). The role of the clinical nurse specialist: Problems and solutions. *Journal of Nursing Administration* 16 (10): 44-48.

52. Rheiner, N.W. (1994). Role theory: Framework for change. In *Contemporary leadership behaviour*, ed., Hein, E.C., & Nicholson, M.J., 307-311. Philadelphia: J.B. Lippincott.

53. Rubin, S. (1988). The expanded role nurse: Role implementation strategies. *Canadian Journal of Nursing Administration* 1 (3): 12-15.

54. Page, N.E., & Arena, D.M. (1991). Practical strategies for CNS role implementation. *Clinical Nurse Specialist* 5 (1): 43-47.

55. Mitchell, A., Patterson, C., Pinelli, J., & Baumann, A. (1995). *Assessment of the need for nurse practitioners in Ontario.* Quality of Nursing Worklife Research Unit. McMaster University/University of Toronto, Working Paper Series 95-7.

Chapter 4

1. Stein, L.I., Watts, D.T., & Howell, T. (1990). The doctor-nurse game revisited. *The New England Journal of Medicine* 322 (8): 546-549.

2. Stein, L.I. (1967). The doctor-nurse game. *Archives of General Psychiatry* 16: 699-703.

3. Salvage, J. (1995). What's happening to nursing? *British Medical Journal* 311: 274-275.

4. Spitzer, W. O., & Kergin, D.J. (1973). Nurse practitioners in primary care. The McMaster University education program. *Canadian Medical Association Journal* 108: 991-995.

5. Spitzer, W.O., Sackett, D.L., Sibley, J.C., Roberts, R.S., Gent, M., Kergin, D.J., Hackett, B.C., & Olynich, A. (1974). The Burlington randomized trial of the nurse practitioner. *The New England Journal of Medicine* 290 (5): 251-256.

6. DeAngelis, C.D. (1994). Nurse practitioner redux. *Journal of American Medical Association* 271 (11): 868-871.

7. Spitzer, W.O., & Kergin, D.J. (1971). The nurse practitioner. Calling a spade a spade. *Ontario Medical Review* 38: 165-166.

8. Mundinger, M. (1994). Advanced-practice nursing-good medicine for physicians? *The New England Journal of Medicine* 330 (3): 211-214.

9. Bradshaw, A. (1995). Nursing and medicine: Cooperation or conflict? *British Medical Journal* 311: 304-305.

10. Brown, S.A., & Grimes, D.E. (1993). *A meta-analysis of process of care, clinical outcomes, and cost-effectiveness of nurses in primary care roles: Nurse practitioners and certified nurseslmidwives.* Washington, DC: American Nurses Association, Division of Health Policy.

11. Dowling, S., Barrett, S., & West, R. (1995). With nurse practitioners, who needs house officers? *British Medical Journal* 311: 309-313.

12. Kletke, P.R., Marder, W.D., & Silberger, A.B. (1984). The growing population of female physicians: Implications for U.S. physician supply. *American Journal of Public Health* 74: 10-13.

13. Marsh, G.N., & Dawes, M.L. (1995). Establishing a minor illness nurse in a busy general practice. *British Medical Journal* 310: 778-780.

14. Ontario Anti-infective Review Panel. (1995). *Anti-infective guidelines for community-acquired infections* 1994/95. Toronto: Ministry of Health.

15. Evans, C.E. (1993). *The Canadian consensus of hypertension management.* The Canadian Hypertension Society.

16. Levine, M., Lexchin, J., & Pellizzari, R. (1995). *Drugs of choice: A formulary for general practice.* Ottawa: Canadian Medical Association.

17. Nolan, M. (1995). Towards an ethos of interdisciplinary practice. *British Medical Journal* 311: 305-307.

18. Zuger, A. (1995). Nurse practitioners in primary care. Letter, *The New England Journal of Medicine* 330 (21): 1539.

19. College of Family Physicians. (1994). *A proposal for a blended funding mechanism.* Unpublished manuscript.

20. Wilson, S. (1995). Report queries savings with doctor-nurse shift. *British Medical Journal* 311: 280.

21. Weinberg, N.L. (1994). Advanced-practice nursing-good medicine for physicians? Letter, *The New England Journal of Medicine* 330 (21): 1536.

22. Ontario Ministry of Health. (1993). *A picture of health: Community health centres in Ontario.*

23. Growe, S.J. (1991). *Who cares: The crisis in Canadian nursing.* Toronto: McClelland and Stewart.

24. Way, D.O., & Jones, L.M. (1994). The family physician-nurse practitioner dyad: Indications and guidelines. *Canadian Medical Association Journal* 151 (1): 29-34.

25. Little, M. (1980). Nurse practitioners/physician relationships. *American Journal of Nursing* 80: 1642-1645.

26. Freedman, B. (April, 1986). The "Team" re-defined. *Canadian Doctor* 8-10.

27. Nurse Practitioners' Association of Ontario. (1993). *Standards of practice for nurse practitioners.* Toronto: Nurses Practitioners' Association of Ontario.

28. Health Disciplines Act, R.S.O. 1990, C.H.4, S.72 (1).

29. Regulated Health Professions Act, 1991, S.O., c.18 (Amended 1993, C.37).

30. Moniz, D.M. (1992). The legal danger of written protocols and standards of practice. *Nurse Practitioner* 17 (9): 58-60.

31. Hoole, A., Greenberg, R.A., & Pickard, C.G. (1988). *Patient care guidelines for nurse practitioners.* (3rd ed.) Boston: Little Brown.

32. Boyton, R.W., Dunn, E.S., & Stephens, G.R. (1983). *Manual of ambulatory pediatrics.* (1st ed.) Boston: Little Brown.

33. Ontario Drug Benefit Formulary. (1995). Toronto: Ontario Ministry of Health.

34. Ontario Ministry of Health. (December, 1994). *Nurse practitioners in Ontario: A plan for their education and employment.* Toronto: Queen's Printer for Ontario.

35. College of Nurses of Ontario. (1995). NP draft regulations. *College Communiqué* 20 (1): 32-34.

36. Health Professions Regulatory Advisory Council. (July, 1995). *Transcript of public forum: Nurse practitioners June 16 and 22.*

37. Health Professions Regulatory Advisory Council. (August, 1995). *Letter to participants regarding nurse practitioner referral.*

38. Gray, C. (1983). Nurse practitioners: Stepping into the doctors' domain. *Canadian Medical Association Journal* 128 (6): 1305-1309.

39. Morgan, P. P., & Cohen, L. (1992). Should nurse practitioners play a larger role in Canada's health care system? *Canadian Medical Association Journal* 146 (6): 1020-1025.

40. Ontario Medical Association. (May, 1995). *Submission to HPRAC on nurse practitioners.*

41. Ontario College of Family Physicians. (May, 1995). *Submission to HPRAC regarding proposed changes to regulations to the scope of nursing practice.*

42. *Response of the College of Physicians and Surgeons of Ontario to HPRAC on the nurse practitioner initiative,* Toronto, May 1995.

43. Mitchell, A., Pinelli, J., Patterson, C., & Southwell, D. (1993). *Utilization of nurse practitioners in Ontario: A discussion paper requested by the Ontario Ministry of Health.* Quality of Nursing Worklife Research Unit. McMaster University/University of Toronto, Working Paper Series 93-4.

44. Ontario Ministry of Health. (November, 1994). *Working together to re-introduce nurse practitioners in Ontario.*

45. Farah, L., Bieda, A., & Shiau, S-YPK. (1996). The history of the neonatal nurse practitioner in the United States. *Neonatal Network* 15 (5): 11-21.

46. National Association of Neonatal Nurses (NANN). Position statement on graduate education for entry into neonatal nurse practitioner practice. *Neonatal Network* 14 (5): 52.

47. Pinelli, J. School of Nursing, Faculty of Health Sciences, McMaster University, Hamilton, Ontario.

48. National Association of Neonatal Nurses. Press Release. (1989). *Advanced practice role definition* (pp. 1-2). Petaluma, CA: National Association of Neonatal Nurses.

49. Ford, L. (1979). A nurse for all settings: The nurse practitioner. *Nursing Outlook* 27: 516-521.

50. Paes, B., Mitchell, A., Hunsberger, M., Blatz, S., Watts, J., Dent, P., Sinclair, J., & Southwell, D. (1989). Medical staffing in Ontario neonatal intensive care units. *Canadian Medical Association Journal* 140: 1321-1326.

5l. Hunsberger, M., Mitchell, A., Blatz, S., Paes, B., Pinelli, J., Southwell, D., French, S., & Soluk, R. (1992). Definition of an advanced nursing practice role in the NICU: The clinical nurse specialist/neonatal practitioner. *Clinical Nurse Specialist* 6 (2): 91-96.

52. Askin, D.F., Bennett, K., & Shapiro, C. (1994). The clinical nurse specialist and the research process. *Journal of Obstetric, Gynecologic, and Neonatal Nursing* 23 (4): 336-340.

53. McGuire, D., & Harwood, D. (1989). The CNS as researcher. In *The clinical nurse specialist in theory and practice*, eds., Hamric, A.B., & Spross, J., 169-198. Toronto: W.B. Saunders.

54. Pinelli, J., & Paes, B. (1995). Advanced practice nurses in neonatal intensive care. In *Recent advances in pediatrics*, ed., David, T.F., VOL 14, 97-107. Edinburgh: Churchill Livingston.

55. Mitchell, A., Watts, J., Whyte, R., Blatz, S., Norman, G.R., Guyatt, G.H., Southwell, D., Hunsberger, M., & Paes, B. (1991). Evaluation of graduating neonatal nurse practitioners. *Pediatrics* 88: 789-794.

56. Mitchell, A., Guyatt, G., Marrin, M., Goeree, R., Willan, A., Southwell, D., Hewson, S., Paes, B., Rosenbaum, P., Hunsberger, M., & Baumann, A. (1996). A control trial of nurse practitioners in neonatal intensive care. *Pediatrics* 98:1143-8.

57. Trotter, C., & Danaher, R. (1994). Neonatal nurse practitioners: A descriptive evaluation of an advanced practice role. *Neonatal Network* 13 (1): 39-47.

58. Schultz, J.M., Liptak, G.S., & Fioravanti, J. (1994). Nurse practitioners effectiveness in NICU. *Nursing Management* 25 (10): 50-53.

59. Carzoli, R.P., Martinez-Cruz, M., Cuevas, L.L., Murphy, S., & Chiu, T. (1994). Comparison of neonatal nurse practitioners, physician assistants, and residents in the neonatal intensive care unit. *Archives of Pediatrics and Adolescent Medicine* 148: 1271-1276.

60. Martin, R.G., Fenton, L.J., Leonardson G., & Reid, T.J.(1985). Consistency of care in an intensive care nursery staffed by nurse clinicians. *American Journal of Diseases of Children* 139: 169-172.

61. Ostrea, E.M., & Schuman, H. (1975). The role of the pediatric nurse practitioner in a neonatal unit. *Journal of Pediatrics* 86 (4): 628-631.

62. DeNicola, L., Kleid, D., Brink, L., Vanstralen, D., Scott, M., Gerbert, D., & Brennan, L. (1994). Use of pediatric physician extenders in pediatric and neonatal intensive care units. *Critical Care Medicine* 22 (11): 1856-1862.

63. Hall, M.A., Smith, S.L., Jackson, J.E., Perks, E.M., & Walton, P. (1992). Neonatal nurse practitioners-a view from perfidious Albion? *Archives of Disease in Childhood* 67 (4 Spec No): 458-462.

64. Way, D.O., & Jones, L.M. (1994). The family physician-nurse practitioner dyad: Indications and guidelines. *Canadian Medical Association Journal* 151 (1): 29-34.

65. Freedman, B. (April, 1986). "The Team" re-defined. *Canadian Doctor*: 8-10.

66. Sackett, D.L., Spitzer, W.O., Gent, M., Roberts, R.S., Hay, W.I., Lefroy, G.M., Sweeny, G.P., Vandervlisd, I., Sibley, J.C., Chambers, L.W., Goldsmith, C.H., MacPherson, A.S., & McAuley, R.G. (1974). A Burlington randomized trial of the nurse practitioner: Health outcomes of patients. *Annals of Internal Medicine* 80: 137-142.

67. Robinson, G., Beaton, S., & White, P. (1993). Attitudes towards practice nurses-Survey of a sample of general practitioners in England and Wales. *British Journal of General Practice* 43: 25-29.

68. Snyder, J.V., Sirio, C.A., Angus, D.C., Hravnak, M.T., Kobert, S.N., Sinz, E.H., & Rudy, E.B. (1994). A trial of nurse practitioners in intensive care. *New Horizons* 2 (3): 296-304.

69. Mitchell, A., Southwell, D., Fram, N., Baumann, A., & Hunsberger, M. Neonatal clinical nurse specialist/nurse practitioner's job satisfaction and impact on the health care team. (In progress).

70. Honigfeld, L., Perloff, J., & Barzansky, B. (1990). Replacing the work of pediatric residents: Strategies and issues. *Pediatrics* 85 (6): 969-976.

71. Michell, A., Pinelli, J., & Southwell, D. (1996). Introduction and evaluation of an advanced nurse practice role in neonatal intensive care. In *Outcome of effective management practice*, ed., Kelly, K., 171-186. California: Sage Publications.

72. Bullough, B. (1992). Alternative models for specialty nursing practice. *Nursing and Health Care* 13 (5): 254-259.

73. Mitchell, A., Pinelli, J., Patterson, C., & Southwell, D. (1993). *Utilization of nurse practitioners in Ontario: A discussion paper requested by the Ontario Ministry of Health.* Quality of Nursing Worklife Research Unit. McMaster University/University of Toronto, Working Paper Series 93-4.

74. Ruth-Sanchez, V., Lee, K.A., & Bosque, E.M. (1996). A descriptive study of current neonatal nurse practitioner practice. *Neonatal Network* 15 (5): 23-29.

75. Buus-Frank, M.E., Conner-Bronson, J., Mullaney, D., McNamara, L.M., Laurizio, V.A., & Edwards, W.H. (1996). Evaluation of the neonatal nurse practitioner role: The next frontier. *Neonatal Network* 15 (5): 31-39.

76. National Association of Neonatal Nurses (NANN): SIG-AP Education Task Force. (1992). *Neonatal nurse practitioners: Standards of education and practice.* Petaluma, California: NANN.

77. National Certification Corporation (NCC) for the Obstetric, Gynecologic and Neonatal Nursing Specialties. *1994/1995 certification program*, 4-5, 36-38. Chicago: NCC.

78. Freund, C.M., & Overstreet, G.A. (1981). The economic potential of nurse practitioners. *Nurse Practitioner* 6: 28-32.

79. Morgan, P.P., & Cohen, L. (1992). Should nurse practitioners play a larger role in Canada's health care system? *Canadian Medical Association Journal* 146 (6): 1020-1025.

80. Lomas, J., & Stoddart, G.L. (1985). Estimates of the potential impact of nurse practitioners on future requirements for physicians in office-based general practice. *Canadian Journal of Public Health* 76: 119-123.

81. Fottler, M.D., Gibson, G., & Pinchoff, D.M. (1980). Physician resistance to manpower innovation: The case of the nurse practitioner. *Social Science Quarterly* 61: 149.

82. Sullivan, J.A., Dachelet, C.Z., & Sultz, H.A. (1978). Overcoming barriers through the employment and utilization of the nurse practitioner. *American Journal of Public Health* 68: 1097.

83. Nichols, L.M. (1992). Estimating costs of underusing advanced practice nurses. *Nursing Economics* 10: 343-351.

84. Pellizzari, R. (1992). *Economic evaluation of the nurse practitioner in primary care delivery.* (Unpublished).

85. Denton, F.T., Gafni, A., Spencer, B.G., & Stoddart, G.L. (1983). Potential savings from the adoption of nurse practitioner technology in the Canadian health care system. *Socio-Economic Planning Sciences* 17 (4): 199-209.

86. American Medical Association. (December, 1993). *Report 35 (1-93) of the Board of Trustees. Economic and quality of care issues with the implications on scopes of practice-physicians and nurses.* Executive summary. Chicago, AMA, 1-30.

87. American College of Emergency Physicians. (June, 1991). *Policy statement. Guidelines on the role of nurse practitioners in emergency departments.* Dallas: ACEP.

88. Atcheson, J. (1991). Medical profession stops nursing practitioners practice. *Alberta Association of Registered Nurses* 47 (9): 10-12.

89. Stoddart, G.L., & Barer, M.L. (1992). Toward integrated medical resources policies for Canada: Remuneration of physicians and global expenditure policy. Canadian Medical Association Journal 147 (1): 33-37.

90. Moore, C.A. (1994). Family physicians and nurse practitioners: Guidelines, not battlelines. *Canadian Medical Association Journal* 151 (1): 19-21.

91. Frew, E.M.S. (1991). The fee-for-service systems should be replaced. *Canadian Medical Association Journal* 145 (7): 763-767.

92. Wright, C.J. (1991). One fee-for-service system should be replaced. *Canadian Medical Association Journal* 144 (7): 900-903.

93. Pearson, L.F. (1993). 1992-1993 update: How each state stands on legislative issues affecting advanced nursing practice. *Nurse Practitioner* 18 (1): 23-37.

94. Chance, G.W. (1989). The crisis in staffing neonatal intensive care units: A taste of things to come? *Canadian Medical Association Journal* 140: 1271-1274.

Chapter 5

1. Registered Nurses Association of Ontario. (December, 1993). *Provincial nurse association applauds move to recognize role of NPs.* Press release.

2. Registered Nurses Association of Ontario. (January, 1994). *Reporting on ... nurse practitioners.* Position Statement.

3. Registered Nurses Association of Ontario. (February, 1994). *RNAO applauds province's commitment to NP.* Press release.

4. Registered Nurses Association of Ontario. (March, 1994). *NP will mean more choice for consumers.* Press release.

5. Registered Nurses Association of Ontario. (February, 1995). *RNs reinforce support for the NP program.* Press release.

6. Registered Nurses Association of Ontario. (May, 1995). *Written submission to HPRAC on referral of nurse practitioners.*

7. Registered Nurses Association of Ontario. (June, 1995). *Submission to HPRAC on referral of nurse practitioners.*

8. Nightingale, F. (1992). *Notes on nursing: What it is and what it is not*, ed., Skvetkowicz, V. London: Scutari Press.

9. Donohue, M. P. (1985). *Nursing: The finest art.* Toronto: C.V. Mosby.

10. Cohen, I. B. (1984). Florence Nightingale. *Scientific American* 250 (3): 128-138.

11. Hektor, L. M. (1994). Florence Nightingale and the women's movement: Friend or foe? *Nursing Enquiry* 1: 38-45.

12. Strong-Boag, V. (1991). Making a difference: The history of Canada's nurses. *Canadian Bulletin of Medical History* 8: 231-248.

13. Woolf, V. (1938). *Three guineas.* London: The Hogarth Press.

14. MacPherson, K. (1990). *Skilled service and women's work: Canadian nursing 1920-1939.* Doctoral Thesis, Simon Fraser University, B.C. (unpublished).

15. Harvey, C. A. (1991). The changing relationship of physicians and nurses. *Canadian Family Physician* 37: 47-50, 225.

16. Hall, D. (1990). *Starting points for reasoning.* Copenhagen, Denmark: Danish Nurses Organization.

17. Spitzer, W. O. (1984). The nurse practitioner revisited: A slow death of a good idea. *The New England Journal of Medicine* 310 (16): 1049-1051.

18. Williams, C. A., & Valdivieso, G. C. (1994). Advanced practice models: A comparison of clinical nurse specialist and nurse practitioner activities. *Clinical Nurse Specialist* 8: 311-318.

19. Smith, M. C. (1995). The core of advanced practice nursing. *Nursing Science Quarterly* 8 (1): 2-3.

20. Watson, J. (1995). Advanced nursing practice ... and what might be. *Nursing and Health Care: Perspectives on Community* 16 (2): 78-83.

21. Nurse Practitioners' Association of Ontario. (1993). *Standards of practice for nurse practitioners.* Toronto: Nurse Practitioners' Association of Ontario.

22. Page, N. E., & Arena, D. M. (1994). Rethinking the merger of the clinical nurse specialist and the nurse practitioner roles. *Image: Journal of Nursing Scholarship* 26 (4): 315-318.

23. Naylor, M. D., & Brooten, D. (1993). The roles and functions of clinical nurse specialists. *Image: Journal of Nursing Scholarship* 25 (1): 73-78.

24. McFadden, F.A., & Miller, M.A. (1994). Clinical nurse specialist's practice: Facilitators and barriers. *Clinical Nurse Specialist* 8: 27-33.

25. Alcock, D. (1994). *The clinical nurse specialist, clinical nurse specialist/ nurse practitioner and other titled nurses in Ontario.* Ontario: Ministry of Health.

26. Schutzenhofer, K. K., & Musser, D. B. (1994). Nurse characteristics and professional autonomy. *Image: Journal of Nursing Scholarship* 26 (3): 201-205.

27. Registered Nurses Association of Ontario. (1994). *Membership statistics.* Toronto: RNAO.

28. Sherwin, S. (1992). *No longer patient: Feminist ethics and health care.* Philadelphia: Temple University Press.

29. Globerman, J. (1990). Free enterprise, professional ideology, and self-interest: An analysis of resistance by Canadian physicians to universal health insurance. *Journal of Health and Social Behaviour* 31: 11-27.

30. Mitchell, A., Patterson, C., Pinelli, J., & Baumann, A. (1995). *Assessment of the need for nurse practitioners in Ontario.* Quality of Nursing Worklife Research Unit. McMaster University/University of Toronto, Working Paper Series 95-7.

31. Mitchell, A., Pinelli, J., Patterson, C., & Southwell, D. (1993). *Utilization of Nurse Practitioners in Ontario: A discussion paper requested by the Ontario Ministry of Health.* Quality of Nursing Worklife Research Unit. McMaster University/ University of Toronto, Working Paper Series 93-4.

32. Griffin, H. M., & Robinson, K.R. (1993). Current procedural terminology (CPT) coded services provided by nurse specialists. *Image: Journal of Nursing Scholarship* 25 (3): 178-186.

33. Ministry of Health. (1994). *Nurse practitioners in Ontario: A plan for their education and employment.* Ontario Ministry of Health.

34. Health Professions Regulatory Advisory Council. (1995). *Transcript of public forum: Nurse practitioners June 16 and 22.*

35. Registered Nurses Association of Ontario. (1994). *Submission to HPRAC on incorporation of physicians and other health care professionals.*

36. Way, D.O., & Jones, L.M. (1994). The family physician-nurse practitioner dyad: Indications and guidelines. *Canadian Medical Association Journal* 151 (1): 29-34.

37. Mahoney, D.F. (1994). The appropriateness of geriatric prescribing decisions made by nurse practitioners and physicians. *Image: Journal of Nursing Scholarship* 26 (1): 41-46.

38 Aitken, L. H., Lake, E.T., Semaan, S., Lehman, H.P., O'Hare, P.A., Cole, C.S., Dunbar, D., & Frank, I. (1993). Nurse practitioner managed care for persons with HIV infection. *Image: Journal of Nursing Scholarship* 25 (3): 172-177.

39. Brown, S.A., & Grimes, D.E. (1993). *Nurse practitioners and certified nurse midwives: A meta-analysis of studies on nurses in primary care roles.* Washington: American Nurses Publishing.

40. Schattschneider, H.J. (1990). Power relationships between physician and nurse. *Humane Medicine* 6 (3): 197-201.

41. Pettengill, M.M., Gillies, D.A., & Clark, C. (1994). Factors encouraging and discouraging the use of nursing research findings. *Image: Journal of Nursing Scholarship* 26 (2): 143-147.

Chapter 6

1. Mason, D.J., & Leavitt, J.K. (1993). Policy and politics: A framework for action. In *Policy and politics for nurses: Action and change in the workplace, government, organizations and community* (2nd ed.), ed., Mason, D.J., Talbott, S.W.,& Leavitt, J. K., 3-17. Philadelphia: Saunders.

2. Presthus, R. (1973). *Elite accommodation in Canadian politics.* Toronto: MacMillan.

3. Dahl, R.A. (1961). Who governs? Democracy and power in the American city. Newhaven, CT: Prentice Hall.

4. Presthus, R. (1991). *Elite accommodation in Canadian politics.* Toronto: Macmillan.

5. Larson, J., & Baumgart, A.J. (1992) Overview: Shaping public policy. In *Canadian nursing faces the future* (2nd ed.), eds., Baumgart, A.J., & Larsen, J., 469-492. Toronto: Mosby.

6. Alcock, D. (1995). *Advanced nursing practice.* Paper presented at the 1995 Nursing Consensus Meeting, Toronto Ontario.

7. Cronenwett, L.R. (1995). Molding the future of advanced practice nursing. *Nursing Outlook* 43 (3): 112-117.

8. Smith, M.C. (1995). The core of advanced practice nursing. *Nursing Science Quarterly* 8 (1): 2-3.

9. Watson, J. (1995). Advanced nursing practice... and what might be. *Nursing and Health Care: Perspectives on Community* 16 (2): 78-83.

10. Mitchell, A., Pinelli, J., Patterson, C., & Southwell, D. (1993). *Utilization of nurse practitioners in Ontario: A discussion paper requested by the Ontario Ministry of Health.* Quality of Nursing Worklife Research Unit. McMaster University/University of Toronto, Working Paper Series 93-4.

11. Pearson, L.J. (1995). Annual update of how each state stands on legislative issues affecting advanced nursing practice. *Nurse Practitioner: The American Journal Of Primary Health Care* 20 (1): 1-27.

12. Health Professions Regulatory Advisory Council. (1995). *Transcript of public forum-Nurse practitioners, June 16 and 22.*

13. Knight Buppert, C. (1995). Justifying nurse practitioner existence: Hard facts to hard figures. *Nurse Practitioner* 20 (8): 43-48.

Chapter 7

1. Department of National Health and Welfare. (1969). *Study of services for Canadian Indians: Summary report.*

2. Department of National Health and Welfare. (1970a). *Report of the committee on clinical training for medical services in the north.*

3. Economic Council of Canada. (1970). *Patterns of growth, (Seventh annual review).* Ottawa: Queen's Printer.

4. Ontario Department of Health. (1970a). *Report of the Ontario Council of Health on health manpower.* (Supplement No.3).

5. Ontario Department of Health. (1970b). *Report of the activities of the Ontario Council of Health.*

6. Ontario Department of Health. (1970c). *Report of the Ontario Council of Health on health care delivery systems.* (Supplement No.5).

7. Haines, J. (1993). *The nurse practitioner: A discussion paper.* Ottawa: Canadian Nurses Association.

8. Boudreau, T.J. (1972). *Report of the committee on nurse practitioners.* Ottawa: Department of National Health and Welfare.

9. LeFort, S. (1978). The nurse practitioner: What happened? *The Canadian Nurse* 74 (4): 13-23.

10. Canadian Nurses Association. (1971). National conference on research in nursing practice. *The Canadian Nurse* 67 (4): 34-40.

11. Dugas, B. (1971). University programs to prepare nurses for an expanded role in Canadian health services. In Boudreau's *Report of the committee on nurse practitioners* (pp.15-36). Ottawa: Department of National Health and Welfare.

12. Allen, M. (1974). Editorial. *Nursing Papers* 9 (2): 2.

13. Canadian Nurses Association and Canadian Medical Association. (1973). *The expanded role of the nurse: A joint statement of CNA / CMA.*

14. *New perspective on the health of Canadians: A working document.* M. Lalonde, Minister of National Health and Welfare. Ottawa: Department of National Health and Welfare, 1974.

15. Ontario Council of Health. (1979). *The nurse practitioner in primary care* (pp.5). Toronto: Queen's Printer.

16. Chambers, L.W. (1979). Financial impact of family practice nurses on medical practice in Canada. *Inquiry* 16: 339-349.

17. Canadian Nurses Association. (1980). *Putting 'health'into health care: A submission to the Hall Health Services Review.*

18. Spitzer, W.O., Sackett, D.L., Sibley, J.C., Roberts, R.S., Gent, M., Kergin, D.J., Hackett, B.C., & Olynich, A. (1974). The Burlington randomized trial of the nurse practitioner The *New England Journal of Medicine* 290 (5): 251-256.

19. Spitzer, W.O., Kergin, D.J., Yoshida, M.A., Russell, W.A., Hackett, B.C., & Goldsmith, C.H. (1973). Nurse practitioners in primary care. The southern Ontario randomized trial. *Canadian Medical Association Journal* 108: 1005-1016.

20. Sackett, D.L., Spitzer, W.O., Gent, M., & Roberts, R.S. (1974). The Burlington randomized trial of the nurse practitioner: Health outcomes of patients. *Annals of Internal Medicine* 80 (2): 137-142.

21. Chambers, L.W., & West, A.E. (1978). Assessment of the role of the family practice nurse in urban medical practices. *Canadian Journal of Public Health* 69: 459-468.

22. Chambers, L.W., & West, A.E. (1978). The St. John's randomized trial of the family practice nurse: Health outcomes of patients. *The International Journal of Epidemiology* 7 (2): 153-161.

23. Fitzpatrick, L. (1978). A nurse practitioner at work. *The Canadian Nurse* 74 (4): 24-27.

24. Boniface, W., & Fry, J. (1978). The primary care nurse: A matter of acceptance. *Ontario Medical Review* 45 (5): 225-228.

25. World Health Organization. (1978). *Primary health care: Report of the international conference on primary health care.* Geneva.

26. *Canada's national-provincial health program for the 1980s: A commitment for renewal.* Emmett M. Hall, Special Commissioner. Ottawa: Department of National Health and Welfare, 1980.

27. *Achieving health for all: A framework for health promotion.* Jake Epp, Chairman. Ottawa: Department of National Health and Welfare Canada, 1986.

28. *Towards a shared direction for health in Ontario: Report of the Ontario Health Review Panel.* J. R. Evans, Chairman. Ottawa: Department of National Health and Welfare.

29. *Health promotion matters in Ontario: A report of the Minister's Advisory Group on health promotion.* S. Podborski, Chairman. Ottawa: Department of National Health and Welfare.

30. *Health for all Ontario: Report of the panel on health goal for Ontario.* R.A. Spasoff, Chairman. Ottawa: Department of National Health and Welfare.

31. Premier's Council on Health Strategy. (1991). *Achieving the vision: Health human resources-Report of the health care system committee.* Toronto: Ontario Ministry of Health.

32. Organization for Economic Co-operation and Development (OECD). (1993). *OCED health systems facts and trends 1960-1991.* Health Policy Studies No. 3. Paris.

33. Health Canada. Health Policy Division. (1994). *National health expenditures in Canada 1975-1993.*

34. Baumgart, A.J. (1992). Evolution of the Canadian health care system. In *Canadian nursing faces the future* (2nd ed.), ed., Baumgart, A.J., & Larsen, J., 35. Toronto: Mosby Year Book.

35. Angus, D.E., Auer, L., Cloutier, J.E., & Albert, T. (1994) *Sustainable health care for Canada.* (Queen's University of Ottawa Economic Projects, 7). Ottawa: University of Ottawa

36. Ontario Economic Council. (1976). *Issues and alternatives, 1976: Health.* Toronto: Ontario Economic Council.

37. Anderson, J.E. (1990). *Public policymaking.* Boston: Houghton Mifflin.

38. Dye, T.R. (1987). *Policy analysis: What governments do, why they do it and what difference it makes.* Birmingham, Al: University of Alabama Press.

39. Stokey, E., & Zeckhauser, R. (1978). *A primer for policy analysis.* New York: WW Norton.

40. Lefort, S.M. (1993). Shaping health care policy. *The Canadian Nurse* 89 (3): 23-27.

41. Ontario Ministry of Health. (1992). *Goals and strategic priorities: Ministry of Health working document.* (Unpub.).

42. Ontario Ministry of Health. (1993). *Partnerships in long-term care-A new way to plan, manage and deliver services and community support.*

43. Ontario Ministry of Health. (1993). *Putting people first: The reform of mental health services in Ontario.*

44. Barer, M.L., & Stoddart, G.L. (1991). *Toward integrated medical resource policies for Canada.* McMaster University. CHEPA Working Paper Series 91-7.

45. Health and Welfare Canada, Health Information Division. (1993). *Historical statistics on active civilian physicians, Canada, the provinces, and the territories 1961-1992.*

46. Barer, M.L., & Stoddart, G.L. (1993). Toward integrated medical resource policies for Canada: Looking back, looking forward. *Canadian Medical Association Journal* 148: 29-32.

47. OCATH/COFM. (1982). *Report of OCATH/COFM Committee for alternatives to residents for patient care.* (UnPub.).

48. Ontario Physician Manpower Data Centre. (1983). *Physician manpower in Ontario.* (UnPub.).

49. Ontario Physician Manpower Data Centre. (1990). *Physician manpower in Ontario.* (UnPub.).

50. Bannerman, H. (1993). Health care reform: More or less for nurses? *Registered Nurse* 5: 14-17, 24.

51. Ontario Ministry of Health. (1995). *Scott, G.W.S. report of the fact finder on the issue of small rural hospital emergency department physician service.* A report commissioned by the Ontario Ministry of Health, Ontario Hospital Association, Ontario Medical Association.

52. *A new approach to rural emergency medical care for small rural hospitals: A report from the Provincial Co-ordinating Committee on Community and Academic Health Science Centre Relations (PCCCAR) Subgroup on human resource issues in the provision of emergency health services in small rural communities.* Dr. J. Rourke, Chairman. Toronto: Ontario Ministry of Health. (UnPub.).

53. PCCCAR Subcommittee on Underserviced Area Needs. (1995). *PCCCAR reports: Equitable health human distribution. Fulfilling underserviced area needs.* Ontario Ministry of Health. (UnPub.).

54. Council of Ontario Faculties of Medicine. (1995). *The Pools framework for managing postgraduate medical education in Ontario.* (UnPub.).

55. Mitchell, A., Pinelli, J., Patterson, C., & Southwell, (1993). *Utilization of nurse practitioners in Ontario: Discussion paper requested by the Ontario Ministry Health.* Quality of Nursing Worklife Research Unit. McMaster University/University of Toronto. Working Paper Series 93-4.

56. Mitchell, A., Patterson, C., Pinelli, J., & Baumann. (1994). *Assessment of the need for nurse practitioners in Ontario.* Quality of Nursing Worklife Research Unit. McMaster University/University of Toronto, Working Paper Series 95-7.

57. Ontario Ministry of Health. (1994). *Nurse practitioners in Ontario. A position paper.* Toronto: Queen's Printer Ontario.

58. Ontario Ministry of Health. (1994). *Nurse practitioner implementation model.* (UnPub.).

59. Ontario Ministry of Health. (1994). *Renewing partnerships in health care: The proposed plan for the education and employment of NPs.* (UnPub.).

60. Ontario Ministry of Health. (1994). *Working together to re-introduce nurse practitioners in Ontario: Summary of the focus groups.* (UnPub.).

61. Ontario Ministry of Health. (1994). *Nurse practitioners in Ontario: A plan for their education and employment.* Toronto: Queen's Printer for Ontario.

Chapter 8

1. Titanich, K., McDonough, J., Woodhead-Lyons, S., & Snell, S. (1996). Back lakes community health pilot project-Alberta, Canada. In *Community as partner: Theory and practice in nursing* (2nd ed.), eds., Anderson, E.T., & McFarlane, J.M. Philadelphia, PA: Lippincott.

2. World Health Organization, Regional Office for Europe. (1984). *Health promotion: A discussion document on the concept and principles.* Copenhagen.

3. World Health Organization. (1978). *Primary health care: Report of the international conference on primary health care,* held in Alma Ata, USSR. Geneva.

4. British Columbia Ministry of Health. (1989). *Healthy communities: The process, a guide for volunteers, community leaders, elected officials and health professionals who want to build healthy communities.*

5. Hampel, D., Richardson, V., & Titanich, K. (1995). *Rainbow Lake: A health communities project.* Presentation to the International Conference on Community Health Centres in Montreal, Quebec.

6. Premier's Commission on Future Health Care for Albertans. (1989). *The rainbow report: Our vision for health.*

7. Government of Alberta. (1991). *Partners in health: The government of Alberta's response to the Premier's Commission on Future Health Care for Albertans.*

8. Barer, M.L., & Stoddart, G.L. (1991). *Toward integrated medical policies for Canada.* McMaster University. CHEPA Working Paper Series 91-7.

9. Alberta Health. Health Planning Secretariat. (1993). *Starting points: Recommendations for creating a more accountable and affordable health system.*

10. Alberta Health. (1993). *Health goals for Alberta: Progress report.*

11. Alberta Health. (1994). *Healthy Albertans living in a healthy Alberta: A three-year business plan.*

12. Regional Health Authorities Act. CR-9.07 (1994).

13. Alberta Health. (1994). *Guidelines for registered nurses in advanced nursing practice providing primary health care services in underserviced communities in Alberta.* Edmonton, AB: Author.

14. Public Health Act and Regulations. CP-27.1 (1984).

15. Alberta Health. (1995). Registered Nurse Providing Extended Health Services Regulation, Alberta Regulation 224/96.

16. Alberta Association of Registered Nurses. (1995). *Competencies for registered nurses providing extended health services in the province of Alberta.* Edmonton, AB: AARN.

17. Ambulance Services Act and Regulations. CA-40.5. (1990).

18. Pharmaceutical Profession Act. CP-7.1 (1998).

19. Athabasca University's Centre for Nursing and Health Studies. (1996). *Advanced graduate diploma in community nursing practice: Proposed curriculum and course outlines.* Athabasca, AB: Author.

20. Health Workforce Rebalancing Committee. (1995). *Principles and recommendations for the regulation of health professionals in Alberta: Final report of the Health Workforce Rebalancing Committee.* Edmonton, AB: Author.

Chapter 9

1. Morris, J.J. (1991). *Canadian nurses and the law.* Toronto Butterworths, 47-48.

2. Bohnen, L. (1994). *Regulated Health Professions Act: A practical guide.* Aurora, Ont.: Canada Law Book, Inc., 11.

3. *Malette v. Schulman.* (1990) 72 0. R. (2nd) 417, 272-273.

4. *Black's Law Dictionary,* (1979) 5th Ed. St. Paul, Minn.: West Publishing Co., pp 215.

5. Ibid p 375.

6. *Regulated Health Professions Act,* 1991, S.O., c. 18 (Amended 1993, c. 37).

7. *Nursing Act*, 1991, S.O. c. 32 {S.11(l)(2).

8. Morris, J. (1991) *Canadian nurses and the law.* Toronto: Butterworths, 44-45.

9. *Ducharme v. Royal Victoria Hospital.* (1940), 69 B. R. 162 (Que.) Affirming 76 C. S. 309.

10. *Chalmers-Francis v. Nelson.* (1936) 6 Cal.(2d) 402, 57 P.(2d) 312.

11. *Frank v. South.* (1917) 175 Ky. 375.

12. *Argonaut Ins. Co. v. Continental Ins. Co.* (1978) 406 N.Y.S.(2d) 96.

13. *Hernicz v. State of Florida.* (1980) Fla. App., 390 So.(3d) 194.

14. *Regulated Health Professions Act*, 1991, S.O. c. 18 (Amended 1993, c. 37) at {27(2).

15. *Nursing Act* (1991), S.O. c. 32,{4.

16. Nursing Act (1991), S.O. c. 32,{5.

17. *The Expanded Nursing Services for Patients Act* S.O. 1997.

18. *Regulated Health Professions Act*, 1991, S.O. c. 18 (Amended 1993, c. 37), {5.

19. Jefferson, C. (June 8, 1995). *Correspondence to participants re: nurse practitioner referral*, Health Professions Regulatory Advisory Council (Ontario).

20. Sellards, S., & Mills, M. (1995). Administrative issues for use of nurse practitioners. *Journal of Nursing Administration* 25 (5): 64-70.

21. College of Nurses of Ontario. (July 1995). When, why and how to use medical directives. *College Communiqué*: 10-14.

22. McGrath, S. (1990). The cost-effectiveness of nurse practitioners. *Nurse Practitioner* 15 (7): 40-42.

23. Hall, J. (1993). How to analyse nurse practitioner licensure laws. *Nurse Practitioner* 18 (8): 31-34.

24. *Black's Law Dictionary*, (1979). 5th Ed. St. Paul, Minn.: West Publishing Co., 930-933.

25. *Dowey v. Rothwell* (1974) 5 W.W.R. 311, 49 D.L.R.3d 82 (Alta. S.C.).

26. *Planned Parenthood of Northwest Ind.*, Inc. v. Vines (1989) 543 N.E.2d 654 (Ind. Ct. App.).

27. *Alef v. Alta Bates Hosp.* (1992). 6 Cal. Rptr. 2d 900. Ct. App 1992.

28. Birkholz, G. (1995). Malpractice data from the national practitioner data bank. *Nurse Practitioner* 20 (3): 32-35.

29. Louisell, D., & Williams, H. (1995) *Medical Malpractice* Vol.1 {3.26 (47), New York: Matthew-Bender.

30. *McDonald v. York Co. Hosp.* (1972). 3 0. R. 469, 28 D.L.R. 3d 521.

31. *Burns v. Owens* (1973) 459 S.W.2d. 303 (Mo.).

32. *Rudeck v. Wright* (1985) 709 P.2d.621 (Mont.).

33. *Malette v. Schulman* (1990) 72 O.R.2d 417 (C.A.).

34. *Reib v. Hughes* (1980) 2 S.C.R. 880, 14 D.D.L.T. 1, 33 N.R. 361, 114 D.L.R. 3d 1.

35. *Consent to Treatment Act*, S.O. 1992, c. 31.

36. *Re Mitchell and St. Michael's Hospital*, (1980) 29 0.R.2d 185, 112 D.L.R.3d 360, 19 C.P.C. 113 (H.C.).

37. *La Fleur v. Cornelis*. (1979). 28 N.B.R. 2d 569 Q.B.

38. *Cahoon v. Franks* (1967) S.C.R. 455.

Notes

a. Personal communication, September 1995, from Dr. Jan Towers, Director of Governmental Affairs, Practice and Research, American Academy of Nurse Practitioners, Washington, U.S.

b. Personal communication, September 1995, from Dr. Jan Towers, Director of Governmental Affairs, Practice and Research, American Academy of Nurse Practitioners, Washington, U.S.

c. Ten Universities in Ontario have developed five courses for the NP educational program. The minimum requirement for the NP role is a nursing degree at a baccalaureate level with the additional NP training. The program includes prior learning assessment.

d. The programs at McMaster University and the University of Alberta prepare NPs at a master's level to perform expanded role functions in neonatal units. The University of Toronto offers a three-month post-master's program which prepares nurses to work in expanded roles in acute care settings.

e. There are approximately 250 nurses that graduated from the NP educational program practising in Canada. In comparison, there are presently 33,000 NPs in the U.S. who have been educated in NP programs.[10]

f. Since all medically necessary health care must occur, by law, within the public health system, government-controlled hospital expansion to some extent constrains a physician's ability to earn income by limiting his or her access to the hospital's limited resources (e.g., operating room time, access to technology such as MRIs, etc.).

g. There have been ongoing discussions and initiatives by Canadian provincial governments to attempt to address maldistribution of physicians.

h. In the U.S., family physicians, general practitioners, general internists, and general paediatricians are considered primary care.[22] In Canada, only general practitioners are considered primary care physicians. With these provisions, there are about 34% primary care physicians in the U.S. compared to 53% in Canada.

i. Personal communication, September 1995, from Dr. Jan Towers, Director of Governmental Affairs, Practice and Research, American Academy of Nurse Practitioners, Washington, U.S.

j. Personal communication, September 1995, from Dr. Jan Towers, Director of Governmental Affairs, Practice and Research, American Academy of Nurse Practitioners, Washington, U.S.

k. Personal communication, December 21, 1995, from Deborah Phillipchuk, Nursing Consultant-Practice and Leanne Dekker, Registrar, Alberta Association of Registered Nurses.

l. Personal communication, December 21, 1995, from Deborah Phillipchuk, Nursing Consultant-Practice and Leanne Dekker, Registrar, Alberta Association of Registered Nurses.

m. Personal communication, December 21, 1995, from Deborah Phillipchuk, Nursing Consultant-Practice and Leanne Dekker, Registrar, Alberta Association of Registered Nurses.

n. There are two other nursing roles in Canada, both with the initials RPN: The Registered Psychiatric Nurse is a non-RN nursing role that exists in the Western provinces of Canada and plays an important role in the care of the mentally ill. The Registered Practical Nurse is a nursing role that focuses on basic technical bedside skills, and as such, practitioners have required additional education to practise in a mental health setting.

o. The reasons for this include fiscal expedience as well as a lack of recognition of, and appreciation for, the full range of knowledge and skills of the professional nurse.

INDEX

A

B

C

D

E

F

G

H

I

L

M

N

O

P

R

Other Publications by New Grange Press

"Let Me Decide"

By Dr. D. W. Molloy

Through age, illness or accidents, people may lose their capacity to understand the nature and consequences of proposed health care decisions. Health care decisions then fall to families, friends and physicians who may not be aware of the patient's wishes and intent.
The health care directive contained in this booklet lets you plan your own future health care in advance. It makes sure your wishes will be known, should there come a time when you can no longer understand your options or communicate your choices to others. Developed over many years of research and consultation, the Let me Decide health and personal care directive.

- Gives each individual the opportunity to choose different levels of treatment according to his or her wishes,
- Helps relieve family and friends of responsibility for decisions in times of crisis
- Guides health care practitioners in making vital decisions when family members are unavailable.
- Has received enthusiastic support from a wide variety of individuals and groups, including doctors, patients, social workers, lawyers, clergy and advocates for the elderly and the disabled.

This booklet is an easy-to follow living Will, written in plain language. It contains clear explanations of treatment options and a sample Directive. Let Me Decide is translated in French, German, Italian, Japanese, Spanish and Swedish which are available on request. Let Me Decide is a complete health care program with three videos:

1. My Health Care - I Decide
2. My Health Care - Understanding My Choices
3. My Health Care - Filling out the Directive

"Train the Trainer" Workshops and lectures are available on request.

Price: $10.00

Standardized Mini-Mental State Examination

~ By Dr. D. W. Molloy

The Folstein mini-mental state examination (MMSE) is the most widely used screening test of cognition in older adults. The Standardized Mini-Mental State Examination (SMMSE) provides clear, explicit administration and scoring guidelines.

The SMMSE takes less time to administer (10.5 minutes) than the MMSE (13.4 minutes). The SMMSE has a significantly lower variability than the MMSE. The intrarater variability is significantly lower with the SMMSE (86%p<0.003) and interrater variance is lower by 76% compared to the MMSE. Intraclass correlation for the MMSE was 0.69 compared to 0.9 for the SMMSE. The SMMSE is now widely used because it is the same as the original Folstein and more reliable.

The SMMSE can be used in the diagnosis and treatment of dementia. It is used to stage the disease, differentiate between the different dementias and assess response to treatment.

Price $5.00

Standardized Mini-Mental State Examination
A User's Guide

~ By Dr. D. W. Molloy

The population is aging. More and more physicians now recognize the importance of cognitive testing in the assessment of older adults. The "Mini-Mental State Examination" is the most widely used screening test of cognitive function in older adults.

This short booklet contains a standardized version of this test, the Standardized Mini-Mental State Examination (SMMSE) and describes how this short test can be used in the diagnosis and treatment of cognitive impairment in older adults. The book describes how the SMMSE is used to stage dementia, assess treatment and develop care plans.

The pattern of changes on the SMMSE provides valuable clues to the cause of cognitive impairment. This short booklet is packed with practical clinical tips, diagnostic aids, tables and figures.

Written by Dr. William Molloy, a Professor of Medicine at McMaster University and Consultant Geriatrician, an expert in the field of dementia for over ten years, this short booklet is a must for health care workers who deal with older adults.

Nurse Practitioners.....The Catalyst of Change

Christine Patterson, Editor

A new nurse practitioner book, complementary to Visions and Voices: The Nurse Practitioner Today, will be available in the fall. Both books are timely and make a significant contribution to outlining how nursing organized itself to realize a vision.

Visions and Voices: The Nurse Practitioner Today is a comprehensive overview of the political, economic and social factors that influence advanced practice roles of nurses.
A number of contributors outline from different perspectives the political process, educational challenges and legal implications of advanced practice. Nurse practitioners discuss their roles and the problems they face in role development. Physicians relate their experiences working with nurse practitioners in primary, secondary and tertiary care settings. This fascinating book provides a unique, detailed account of the challenges faced by professional nursing in health care.

This second book describes the progress made with the nurse practitioner initiative across Canada and documents the struggles faced by the nursing profession as it tries to define and redefine the role of nurses in health care restructuring. Some provinces have embraced the nurse practitioner role while others attempt to develop alternate models. The perspectives of the professional bodies in the provinces and territories of Canada and the emerging professional, legal and practice issues emanating from this movement are an important part of this book.

While not all are in agreement the nurse practitioner role is the best approach in their situation, there is agreement for the advancement of nursing's role in the health care system.

Price $20.00

Crabtee's Riddle
by Joanne Patterson

"Crabtee's Riddle", the first volume of a three part trilogy "The Wheel of Fortune", is a white knuckle page-turner, each new twist plunging the reader deeper and deeper into a fantastic labyrinth of spiritual high jinks, intrigue and mystery. The story is full of crystal balls, Tarot cards, wizards, ghosts, prophesies, past life regressions, wound into a brilliant mysterious adventure as the heroines Sally and Iris hang on gallantly to the Wheel of Fortune for the ride of their life

The world of Iris O'Connoll starts to spin one night and it never stops. Iris discovers her mysterious connection with the tarot card, The Wheel of Fortune, when she was fleeing a romantic betrayal. Desmond Rathbone, the arcane tarot reader reveals to her the mystery of a crystal ball handed down to him by his grandmother. Desmond challenges Iris to face her own destiny and dares her to pick a card that most closely resonates with her life. She picks the Wheel of fortune and after that, nothing stays the same. The hectic, spinning, spiritual adventure is filled with fear, adventure and enlightenment. Spooked by her best friend Sally's ominous dream she had of tunnels, warnings and past life redemption, they flee to the Northern town of Heather where life explodes into new and mysterious conundrums. Each time Iris thinks she has escaped, the wheel throws her into another dimension full of predicaments, excitement and surprises.

A business card stuck to her shoe leads to Astrid, the intriguing proprietor of the Oracle bookstore and soul artist. She learns about a notorious book hidden in her attic. Iris meets the author, Charles Crabtree who has been dead for many years. Crabtree's "Book of Predictions" contains prophetic insights for the year 2000 to 3010 and ends with a cryptic and mysterious riddle. Iris and Sally set out on an exciting, and at times harrowing adventure to unravel this riddle.

Iris encounters Merlin the wizard who borrows her body in a bone chilling experience. Iris and Sally are out of their depth in this strange and fascinating world, lunging from one adventure to the next as the wheel spins them closer and closer to an appreciation of the riddle's importance.

Joanne Patterson lives in Bracebridge, Ontario and has received an Honours degree in History from McMaster University, Hamilton. Joanne is a poet who practices alternative therapy and has independently studied spirituality for more than ten years. "Crabtree's Riddle" is the first volume of "The Wheel of Fortune" trilogy.

Price $20.00

"Capacity to Decide"

By Dr. D. W. Molloy, Dr. P. Darzins, Dr. Strang

Capacity to Decide is a short, comprehensive book which describes a new six-step capacity assessment to measure decision-specific capacity, with clear instructions on its use. This book describes how this new assessment process process can be applied to measure capacity for:

- personal care,
- health care,
- property and finances,
- advance directives,
- Wills and Powers of Attorney
- driving
- sexuality and intimacy

There are literally hundreds of helpful hints for interviewing and dealing with issues such as depression, delusions, denial in the assessment process. You will learn how to deal with different thresholds of understanding and idiosynchratic values and beliefs. Other topics covered include driving, sexuality and intimacy.

This process has been developed during consultation with literaly hundreds of professionals, including doctors, nurses, physiciatrists, financial advisors, real estate agents, accountants, lawyers, social workers, occupational therapists, physiotherapists and lay people. It has been applied widely in clinical practice, in the assessment of a wide range of individuals whose capacity was challenged.

"Capacity to Decide" is practical guide and an invaluable tool for health care workers, members of the legal profession and anyone who needs to measure capacity in patients or clients. This process has also been used widely in the court system, where decisions about on capacity are in dispute. "Capacity to Decide", has many figures, tables and charts describing decisional aids which are used in the process.

It is written for professionals and laypersons. This book is a "must" for anyone who deals with clients or patients whose capacity may be called into in question.

Price $24.00

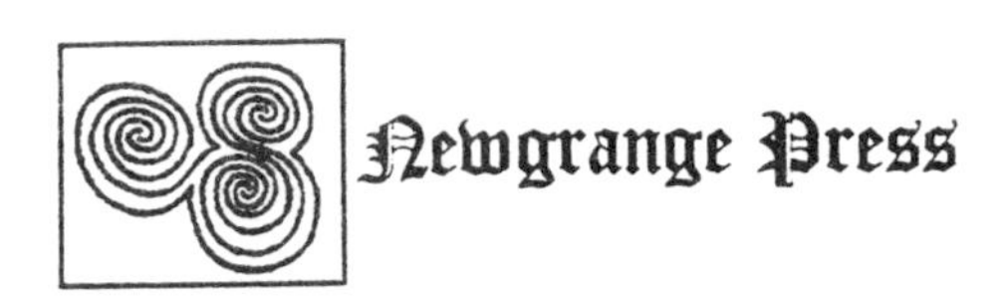

For more information or to order, write to:

Newgrange Press
428 Orkney Road
R.R.1 Troy, Ontario
Canada L0R 2B0

Tel: (905) 628 0354
Fax: (905) 628 4901
e-mail: idecide@netcom.ca
website: www.netcom.ca/~idecide

Newgrange Press U.S.A.
6600 Harrod's View Circle
Prospect, K.Y. 40059

Newgrange Press (Ireland)
The Stables, Woodstown,
Waterford, Ireland

Tel: 353 51 870152
Fax: 353 51 871214

Newgrange Press (Australia)
PO Box 7077
Shenton Park
W Aust 6008

Tel: 08 9346 8107
Fax: 08 9346 8232
email:clarnett@medeserv.com.au

Newgrange Press (Japan)
100-1, Kashiyama,
Habikino, Osaka
(583-0886), Japan

Tel: 81 729 542000
Fax: 81 729 547560

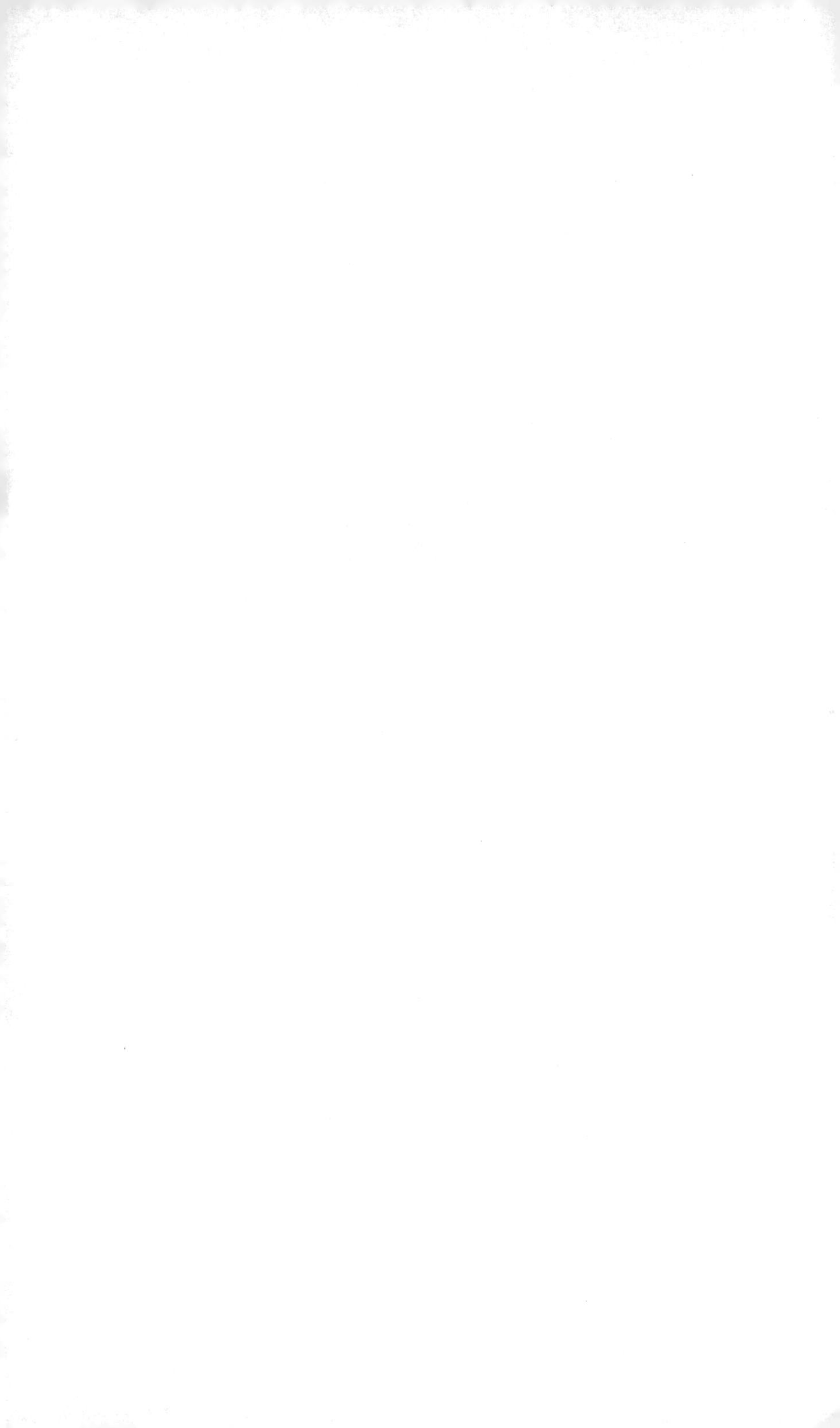